# *V!*

## *A Love Letter to Every Woman and Girl*

### *A Comprehensive Guide to Understanding Vulvovaginal Health*

*Dr. TaMara R. Griffin*

Cover design: Quan Ollie
Editor: FaLessia Booker

## Disclaimer:

This is not designed to be a "be all, end all" comprehensive sex book. It is designed to provide the reader with basic information regarding sexual health in a fun, educational, and entertaining manner. This book is not designed to diagnose or replace the professional assessment of a clinician. For more in depth information, counseling, or therapy regarding sexual concerns (i.e., health, dysfunctions, diseases etc.) please contact your primary physician, mental health clinician, sex therapist, or sexologist. You may also contact Dr. TaMara Griffin. If you feel you are experiencing a mental health or medical emergency, put this book down immediately and call 911, your medical or mental health provider, and/ or go to your local hospital.

*V!* is grounded in more than 15 years of my academic research from studying women and girl's beliefs attitudes and behaviors regarding their bodies and their sexuality. It is also based on over 20 years of personal and professional experiences, as well as stories from the beautiful women and girls that I have worked with and counseled.

# DEDICATION

## A Love Letter to Every Woman and Girl

My Beloved,

*V!* is dedicated to you! We were created as beautiful beings! I pray that we learn to understand, honor, embrace, and celebrate our bodies! I pray that as we learn to respect our bodies, we increase the value of who we are and reduce our risk for sexually transmitted infections and HIV. We hold the power! Our bodies are a temple—let us treat it as such!

With all my love,

Dr. TaMara

# ACKNOWLEDGMENTS AND THANKS

First and foremost, ALL glory and praises belong to the Most High! The Almighty! My Alpha and Omega, my Beginning and Ending, and the Author and the Finisher of my story — God! Thank you Father, for blessing me and choosing me to share this powerful and life-saving message with Your people. Father, I pray that You continue to use me and allow me to share this message of healthy sexuality until my very last breath. How dare I not? Father, our people are perishing from a lack of knowledge. May the work that I do continue to be a blessing to the lives of others. Help them to understand the direct and indirect consequences of their sexual choices. Help them to understand the power and the responsibility of their sexuality. Lastly Father, help them to make safer and healthier informed decisions regarding their sexuality. In Jesus' name, Amen.

I would like to acknowledge and thank the following people for their unwavering support and encouragement they have given me throughout the years. First and foremost, I would like to say thank you to my mother and father, Clarence and Bettina Campbell. When your 13 year old daughter said she wanted to be a sex therapist, you did not shut her down; instead, you helped her to make sense of what it really meant. I thank you for that! Daddy, no matter how much I talk about sex, I will always be your little girl! Momma, in so many ways I am just like you! And I would not have it any other way. You have taught me so much. I am so blessed to have you and Daddy! Thank you for supporting and nurturing all my dreams. But most importantly, thank you for being praying parents and teaching me the importance of having a relationship with God.

I would like to thank Quan Ollie for the amazing cover design. You guys rock! For the second time, you have captured my vision perfectly. It is always such a pleasure to work with you both. You have a gift. I pray that God increases your portion.

I have to thank my amazing editor, FaLessia Booker! You did such an awesome job! Your comments and feedback helped to bring my dream to fruition! I could not have done it without you! You were invaluable and I thank you for the bottom of my heart!

I am sending much love and many blessings to all the amazing men and women who have shared their personal stories with me. Thank you for entrusting me with the most sacred and vulnerable parts of your life! With all that I am, I thank you for all your support, encouragement and kind words over the years! It is because of you that I am able to do the work that I do. You inspire me! I honor, uplift, and thank you!

Last but not least, I thank my husband, Marvin L. Griffin. Thank you, for understanding just how much this human sexuality thing means to me. You love me unselfishly and unconditionally, and for that I am eternally grateful!

# Table of Contents

# INTRODUCTION

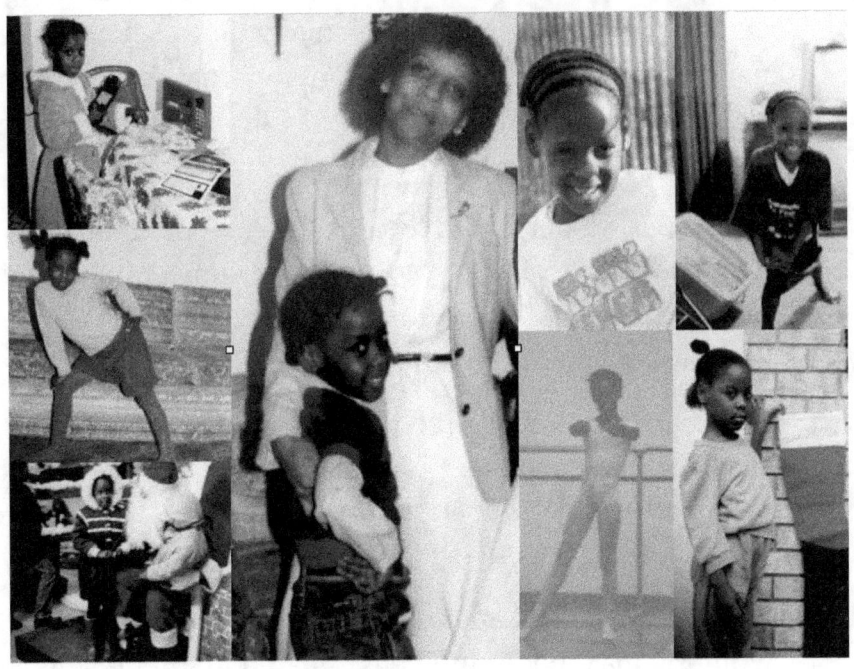

## THE "TALK"
*I was nine! Yup...NINE!*

My mom was always very open and honest about sex—
sometimes a little too much! However, what I truly
appreciate about my mom is that she rarely held back—she
talked to me in a very age-appropriate way so that I could
understand what she was saying.

Circa 1981: A nine-year-old girl sits on her bed in her
bedroom, playing with her baby dolls and getting ready for

bed. It was a night I would never forget—little did I know, this night would change my life forever...

My mom entered my room. In her hand was the purple *Childcraft* #15 encyclopedia and a bag of "stuff" which I had never seen before. What could she want? Now I had already peeked in that book many times before, so I knew (with a very basic understanding) that that book was all about big kid "stuff," so why was she coming in my room with that book in her hand?

Seeing a perplexed look on my face, my mother must have sensed my confusion because she immediately stated that I had done nothing wrong. "I just want to talk to you about where babies come from."

Immediately, I remembered that not too long ago, I had asked her this same question, and now my mom felt the need to answer. Equipped with all her armor, she began to explain.

As she talked about menstrual cycles, vaginas, "wombs," maxi pads, and belts, I stared in utter disgust. As if the "talk" wasn't bad enough, she had the nerve to demonstrate how to use a doggone sanitary belt! I remember thinking, "Enough already! Enough!" All I wanted to do was play with my baby dolls.

Although my mom was always sex-positive and very open and honest about sexuality, she left out definitely some things! I know you're probably thinking, "What in the heck could she have possibly left out? She covered periods, pads, belts, bras, crushes, consequences, and chocolate! My God, how I do love chocolate...(see my book *I AM Sex* for more about my love for chocolate!)

Actually, there were many things she left out, and I'm sort of glad she did, because I think talking about sexual positions that her and my dad used could have been very traumatic and ruined my images of sex forever. So in that sense, I'm very grateful that she left some things out! Even now…the visual…ugh, never mind!

Hey, that might actually be a great method of birth control for some kids! Imagine mom and dad walking in the rooms saying to their kids, "We just had some amazing sex! Wanna hear all about it?" I don't know about ya'll, but that might have just ruined everything for me!

Nevertheless, while I'm very grateful for what she did tell me, I am more grateful for the things I learned on my own) i.e. orgasms, female ejaculation and sex toys…OH MY!!!)

Whew! OK…bring it back!

I know my experience may have been unique. Many other young girls and even some women were not blessed enough to have someone to talk to about the "birds and the bees," and as a result, they were left to learn about their bodies from their friends, television, books, magazines or whatever they could get their hands on. As a result, many women have not received appropriate sex-positive information, which has left them feeling sexually inadequate, misinformed and unprepared to have a sex-positive experience and positive sex-esteem, which may have caused them to put themselves at risk and/or in compromising situations and even conform to some unhealthy sexual images that have been perpetuated by the media.

Unfortunately, lack of proper education and resources contribute to, and even shape, views regarding sexuality. In many ways, it is also the culprit behind the "down there" detachment or disassociation from our bodies, which leads women to talk about their bodies as some separate entity apart from who they are. It also helps to contribute to the sexual dysfunction and negative and unhealthy ways in which we view our sexualities.

## THE REASON

*"My pussy that fi-yah!"* a young lady excitedly exclaimed while snapping her fingers and rolling her neck in all her grandeur!

Not too long ago, I was chatting with a group of young women about their thoughts on their bodies and sexual empowerment. Many of the girls in the group were of the belief that sexual empowerment was all about the "pussy." The consensus of the group was, "I have a pussy; I can have sex; therefore, I am empowered," "I can please my man," "My baby daddy keeps coming back to me over all his other baby mamas, so I must be doing it right," "My pussy that wet-wet," or "I'm wearing my 'freakum' dress to the club, 'cause I know they want me."

As I listened to these beautiful young women laugh, sometimes roll their eyes and in many ways, embrace the images of hyper-sexualized women in the media, i.e., "video chicks," "girls on TV," "reality chicks," etc., I was not at all surprised—these are the images that our young women aspire to. These are the images that they identify with because after all, "they the ones who getting the men and the money cause they boss bitches!"

*Now whose fault is this:*

- the media for their portrayal of women and girls bodies?
- generational patterns that passed down from great-grandma to mama?
- social determinants that are unique to communities or color?
- schools for their lack of comprehensive sex education?
- churches for failing to talk about healthy sexuality from a moral and public health standpoint?
- politicians for pushing their abstinence-only agenda, (that is, until it involves their child)?
- institutions that create systemic barriers that make it hard for women and girls to access the education, prevention, and care services they so desperately need?

The list goes on, but regardless of where we decide to point the finger and place the blame, the fact of the matter is that *we* have failed *them*! We are losing too many of our young women and girls to unintended consequences of their sexual choices. Now we have to accept the responsibility — what we have swept under the rug, kept hidden behind closed doors, or remained tight-lipped about for so long is now walking out of our doors, scantily clad in tight clothing, wearing high heels and operating under the belief that just because she has a pussy, she's sexually empowered.

*What do we do?*

Break the cycle! Have the conversation!

From that conversation, *V!* was born! I left that group knowing that there was still so much more work to do! I left that group affirmed that my message of healthy sexuality and sexual empowerment was needed more than ever; and not just for young women, but for *all* women. We have been so brainwashed about sexuality that we are lost — perhaps by no fault of our own, but nevertheless lost. Many of us have never had the conversation. Many of us just simply do not know because we have not been taught or told anything different. Therefore, I must continue to remain at the forefront of the conversation. I refuse to idly stand by and watch our women, young and old, continue to make poor choices regarding their sexuality when I can do something about it! I refuse to let anyone stifle my voice! I'm about the business of saving lives — if you're not, then move out of the way, because you are part of the problem. Please kindly step aside and let me do the work!

Having a pussy does not make you sexually empowered! It simply means that...you have a pussy (or, shall I say, a vagina!) That's it!

## MY BELOVED! THIS IS FOR YOU!

I wrote *V!* for every woman and girl who did not or do not have a resource to learn about one of the most beautiful, powerful and precious thing in this world — the *V!* — the way my mother educated me and conveyed it in a way that it made sense!

I also wrote *V!* to empower women and girls with the knowledge, skills, and tools to make safer and healthier decisions regarding their sexuality. I want to teach them how to advocate for themselves so that they will not feel ashamed, embarrassed, or belittled. I wanted them to love themselves and their bodies. I wanted them to celebrate their sexuality, but most importantly, I want them to be proud of who they were as women and girls.

Finally, I wrote *V!* to help women and girls learn to advocate for themselves. Given the negative practices that many of my family members and friends have experienced at the hands of physicians that lack cultural humility, competency, or bedside manner, it became personal! I made it my mission to talk to and empower women and girls so they would not have to have damaging experiences.

Because of this, I devoted myself to empowering women and girls to discover, explore, understand, celebrate, honor, and embrace our bodies: our *V!*

## SO, WHAT IS *V!?*

*V!* is the culmination of my journey through the field of human sexuality over the past 20 years. On the pages of this book, you will find funny personal stories, sensual poetry, educational information, tips, tools, and skills that will help you understand, respect, celebrate, and embrace your body.

*V!* is a discussion, a frame of reference for every woman, girl, grandmother mother, sister, daughter, aunt, and cousin! On the pages of V, you will find yourself. Whether you are a single mom, married a housewife, college student, professional career working woman or a young girl trying to understand her body, there is something on these pages for you. It doesn't matter whether you are a virgin, sexually experienced, or sexually repressed; there is something on these pages for you. Black or white, yellow or green, there is something on these pages for you.

*V!* was written to break the cycle of negative, unhealthy intergenerational patterns that have been passed down from great-grandma, to grandma, to mom and to daughters. *V!* is an attempt to undo and dispel all the unhealthy and negative messages that women and girls have received about their over the years. It is also designed to create a healthy self-esteem and sex-esteem and to give women permission to understand, love, respect, and appreciate our bodies!

*V!* is a book containing all the wonderfully amazing things about our beautiful bodies — some of which your mother never told you about (well, unless you had a mother like mine, that is!) While I am certainly not the first person to write a book on vulvovaginal health, I am the first to write about how our vulvovaginal health is tied to every dimension (mental, emotional, spiritual, financial, social, biochemical, energetical, institutional, legal, political, and physical) of our life. I hope that this book will challenge you to learn information and ideals, to make different choices, to ask probing questions, and to take steps to fully understanding, celebrating, honoring, and embracing your *V!*

# IF YOUR VULVA COULD TALK, WHAT WOULD IT SAY?

*"Down there," "you know… that," "it," "or "this area," some of the vague or slang expressions we use when referring to or speaking about our vulva and vaginas. The sometimes seemingly awkward nature in which we talk about our vulva and vaginas, gives the impression that it's some deep, dark, mysterious black hole or something. We are so embarrassed by and disconnected from our genitalia that that we don't even associate it part of our own body. And why is that?*

*There are many reasons women disassociate themselves from owning the beauty of the genitalia; some of which date back to slavery. In addition the messages we receive from media, family, friends and even ourselves regarding women's vulva and vaginas, are not always the most empowering. Not to mention, some are even over sexualized and downright degrading. Society perpetuates the belief that the vulva and vagina is this dirty thing that needs to be cleansed of its filth, as evident by all the feminine hygiene products on the market. There are even cosmetic procedures to "pretty up" the ugly disgusting vulva. Constantly being inundated with such messages, how does one not hold a shameful view of the genitalia? It's beliefs, attitudes and feelings like these that contribute to the unhealthy behaviors that put women at risk for HIV and other sexually transmitted infections, victimization, abuse, body image issues, unhealthy relationships, mental health challenges and so much more.*

*When was the last time we grab a mirror and looked at your vulva; touching and exploring its delicate and intricate folds? How many times have we actually taken the opportunity* to get to know our vulva and vagina? If you could have a conversation with your genitalia, what would she say? Would it be a reunion between happy old friends or a bittersweet greeting of strangers on the street? Would there be an exchange of pleasantries or apologies? If another one of your friends happened to walk in on the conversation, would you be embarrassed to introduce her or would you be proud of her feminine power and beauty? If she asked you the question, can you honestly say you took good care of her all these years? Or would she burst into tears because you disassociate yourself from her because of the fear, shame, stigma, judgment, trauma and disrespect you allowed her to endure from others?

It's time for a shift. We must begin to break those negative intergenerational patterns and disempowering media messages that contribute to a lack of SEX-esteem when it comes to our genitalia. Just as no two women are alike, no two vulvas and vaginas are alike; they are just as unique as each of us! It's important to become intimately acquainted with our bodies. Not just the correct terminology and function but also understanding the power and connection to all the dimensions of sexuality. We must to learn to value, embrace, honor and celebrate all of our womanhood. For our vulva and vagina are the doors of life and also a means of providing pleasure, how could we not respect its power, purpose and beauty!

Apologize this moment for any lack of respect, love and appreciation! It time to make things right and allow her to reclaim her rightful place right now!

My Beloved, trust and believe you are not the only one who may have well..not been as loving as you could have to your vulva/vagina. I am sure that many of us, including myself, have not always made the best decisions when it come to who *and/or what we have allowed into our most sacred space nor have we always been a conscientious judge of the messages that we have received about, you know...."down there." However, the beautiful thing about it is that we do not have to continue to bear the burden of our mishaps and the shame that has become us. We have the opportunity to make amends with ourselves and our bodies from this very moment. We have been given the permission to forgive, heal and reshape our views on our vulvas and vaginas!*

# CHAPTER 1:

# IT'S TIME TO ADDRESS SHAME

Given the historical context and social construction of women and girl's bodies and sexuality, it is important to move forward, reclaim, and redefine our images in a way that does not cause us to compromise our integrity or continue to shame us. And for heaven's sake, let us stop disguising the use of our bodies as some alternative form of empowerment that only perpetuates the bureaucracy of a society who is feeding us all these distorted ideals; ideals which are set by those who objectify, diminish, disregard and shame women and girls bodies.

> *"We've chosen, consciously or subconsciously, to PLACE our vulvovaginal health at risk over the years because of the shame that society has placed on the value of women's bodies." — Dr. TaMara*

## WHAT IS SHAME?

Shame is a harmful emotion that can result from the comparison of self to societal ideals, behaviors, and standards. The comparison can be self-inflicted or forced on us by others. Shame is about fear, secrecy, silence, and judgements. When we experience any or all of those four things, we experience shame. Unfortunately, we live in a society that in many ways support shaming messages. We are taught to embody these messages. In many ways, we become these messages in a dire effort to "fit in." with the status quo. If we do not adopt these messages (for whatever reason), we are shamed even further. When we are full of shame, we are more likely to engage in self-destructing behaviors that put us at risk for mental, emotional, social, financial, spiritual, physical risks. In addition, we are more likely to attach and/or shame others.

## WHY DO WE HAVE SHAME?

Stolen women, we are still perpetuating the behaviors that have been ingrained in us, some of which predate slavery. We continuously allow the society and the media to capitalize on our bodies as if we are still nothing more than objectified erotic capital. In many ways, the sexual images that represent women in the media as hyper-sexualized jezebel place us -right back on the auction block or master's house -for sale disguised as entertainment. Somehow, in our minds and in the minds of others, these degenerative images of women have become the defining factor for women's bodies and sexuality.

## WHAT DOES SHAME LOOK LIKE?

Shame has many faces including, but not limited, to:

- self-doubt
- low self-esteem
- low self-efficacy
- substance abuse

- self-harm
- addiction
- suicide
- depression
- embarrassment
- perfectionism
- overly critical
- anxiety
- isolation
- engaging in risky sexual behaviors

## THE CREATION OF SHAME

> *"We spend a lifetime trying to distance ourselves from our body because we feel like we don't fit in. We do not feel worthy because of the shame that we have experienced throughout the course of our lives. Our sense of worthiness is an important piece that gives us access to love and acceptance of ourselves. In order to begin to develop a sense of worthiness, we must understand the creation of shame and begin to address it." — Dr. TaMara*

Shame is created from a variety of ways from many sources. Some you may already be familiar with, while others may have never even crossed your mind. So where do shaming messages come from? Where do we place the blame? Do we blame generations of patterns that have been passed down? Do we blame the social determinants that are unique to communities or color? Do we blame churches, faith organizations, or spiritual leaders for failing to provide a safe space to have open and honest conversations about women and girls bodies? Do we blame politicians for pushing their abstinence-only agenda, that is, until it becomes their child; or do we blame institutions that create these systemic barriers that make it hard for individuals to access the education, prevention and care services they so desperately need? Do we blame society and the media for their hyper-sexualized messages that bombard social media, the internet, entertainment and the music industry?

The list goes on and on, but regardless of where we decide to point the finger and place the blame, the fact of the matter is that women and girls are bombarded with shaming messages about our bodies. In order to effective address shame, we must first understand *how* shame is created, *where* it comes from, and *what* impact it has so that you can consciously and actively deal with them.

*Intergeneration patterns and behaviors*: Passed down from generation to generation, unhealthy negative patterns, behaviors and beliefs are like viruses replicating and spreading from one family member to another, infecting our thought patterns and becoming deep-rooted within the subconscious mind. As young girls, we learned about ourselves from what we were taught and exposed to (or not exposed to) by our mothers, who learned from her mother, who learned from her mother, and so on. If our mother did not know how to be empowered, it would have been next to impossible for her to teach her daughter how to be an empowered woman. This is not an attempt to place blame on mothers, but a way to help identify some of the behavior patterns that contribute to the circumstances you may face today. Because you have not been taught and do not know any differently, you will continue to make the same mistake until you identify the dangerous, negative, cyclical behaviors and commit to changing them. You are not obligated to fulfill the destiny dictated to you through kinship. You can decide **at this very moment** to break the negative cycle by reprogramming your thoughts, beliefs, and behaviors. By doing so, you begin to chart a new course, you can change destiny for yourself as well as for future generations of women within your family.

*The "Good Girl" Guilt.* Good girls don't! Many girls receive this message growing up. While intended to prevent girls from engaging in sex or certain sexual behaviors, this heavy judgment-laden message helps to birth shame about the body and sexuality. When we categorize sex as something that only bad girls do, we subconsciously send the message that "good" girls should not enjoy sex. The challenge that this creates is that as our "good" girls grow up and become women who get married, and still are harboring the "good girls don't" stigma. As a result, they are less likely to experience sexual pleasure with their partner, which can ultimately contribute to significant problems in their relationship. In addition, many girls who grow up with this belief may suffer from sexual dysfunction that may have been prevented if they grew up with a healthy view of sexuality. In addition, this belief reinforces the shame and stigma surrounding our bodies and our sexuality. The negative consequences of this are that as our girls grow up and become women, they tend to be less likely to have healthy and positive feelings regarding their body and their sexuality. We need to equip our girls with the truth so they can not only love their bodies, but also protect themselves and embrace and own their sexuality.

***Societal Beliefs, Cultural Norms, and Standards:*** Ever-changing social beliefs, cultural norms, and expectations influence women and girls experience their bodies. Each society and cultural has different beliefs, norms and standards about sexuality that serves as a framework for the conceptualization of women and girls bodies. Different cultures vary concerning beliefs, norms, and standards. Exploring cultural influences provides a critical lens for understanding how culture affects an individual's thoughts, beliefs, attitudes, and values on women and girls bodies. What may be considered or deemed as acceptable in one culture may be considered very offensive and/or unacceptable in another. The relationship that a society or culture has with sexuality–whether healthy or unhealthy–can have a profound impact on women and girls bodies.

***Media:*** Media serves to perpetuate a number of social scripts and conceptual frameworks about sexuality. Sex is visible in all forms of media: the World Wide Web, magazines, movies, and music continue to shape societies thoughts, beliefs, and attitudes regarding what is considered appropriate or "normal" when it comes to sexuality. TV programs such as Love *& Hip Hop*, *The Real Housewives*, and *The Bachelorette* are filled with the same old script: images regarding women and girls bodies and sexuality. These images and ideologies continue to have an effect on people's developing sexual identities and sexual attitudes towards women and girls bodies. In addition, they help to add to the layers of intergenerational patterns, stigma, shame, guilt, and embarrassment surrounding women and girls. Unfortunately, our society has become desensitized to seeing such images. The unfortunate and damaging impact is that these images and ideologies have become so embedded in our psyche that if we are not careful, they ultimately become our reality.

*Religion/Spirituality/Faith:* There is a critical need for sexuality education among faith communities. However, because of negative religious, legalistic, and moral attitudes about behaviors associated with sexuality, many faith organizations are reluctant to address concerns regarding sexuality. Unfortunately, this antiquated ideology helps to contribute to behaviors that put individuals at risk for sexually transmitted infections (STIs) and HIV.

Historically, faith organizations have been the foundation of the community, a vehicle for dissemination, and a conduit for providing social services for their congregants and the surrounding community. Faith organizations are a place that people trust and turn to in their time of need for healing and support. Given the fact that faith, spirituality, and religious beliefs are such an important aspects of many people's lives, it is extremely important to provide faith leaders with the knowledge, skills, and tools needed to make their organizations safe, supportive, and non-judgmental space where their congregants can have conversations about women and girls bodies.

***Unspoken Messages:*** In many ways, what adults model to children can have a significant impact on their choices they make, worldview, and behavior. The unspoken messages from adults regarding their bodies are oftentimes more powerful than their spoken messages in shaping children's perception of their bodies. Some forms of unspoken messages include body language, facial expressions, touch, eye contact, and the actions of looking while talking and listening, clothing, etc. Not having conversations about our bodies sends an unspoken message that it is taboo and something that should not be talked about. It teaches girls "do not ask, do not tell." This is a very dangerous unspoken message to send, because it puts them at risk for unintended consequences of sexuality. It also teaches them to keep quiet should they find themselves in a potentially dangerous situation. Finally, it teaches them not to come to you if they have questions about their bodies.

## Undoing the Damage and Overcoming Body Shame
*So, how do we move from shame to empowerment?*

*"Only when we are brave enough to explore the darkness will we begin to discover our light."*
*-Dr. TaMara*

Overcoming shame requires courage, vulnerability and audacity because it focuses us to dig deep and face our imperfections, fears, doubts, unfounded beliefs, attitudes, and behaviors. You know all the "-ish" that we've been struggling with and/or running from. When we dig deep, we develop authenticity. Authenticity is a daily practice of letting go of who others and we think we are supposed to be and embracing who we really are. Authenticity isn't always the *safe* or *popular* option, but it is the *necessary* option. Shame loses power when we address it. One of the most dangerous things to do after a shaming experience is to bury our shame in secrecy. When we bury our shame, it begins to fester and grow. Shame hates it when we confront it because it begins to empower us. In order to overcome shame, we have to be willing to recognize shame, look it in the face, and identify healthy, intentional, restorative ways to move through it. That begins with having an empowered consciousness.

### What is an empowered consciousness?

Empowered consciousness is a daily way of living that enables you to be completely authentic to who you are by actively addressing shame and choosing love.

**Em ·pow ·ered** Transitive verb:
em ·pow ·ered , em ·pow ·er ·ing , em ·pow ·ers

Empowered refers to increasing the spiritual, emotional, social, intellectual, physical, and financial wellness of an individual and their environment. It often involves the developing self-esteem and belief in one's own capacities. According to *Wikipedia*, the free encyclopedia, empowerment is driven ultimately by the individual's belief in their capability to influence events in and around their lives.

The process of living an empowered life means listening to your inner voice, regardless of the pressure of family, friends, group belief systems, and society at large — trusting yourself enough to believe that you know what is best for you.

In addition, living an empowered life allows you to gain the knowledge, skills, beliefs, and attitudes needed to effectively deal with the changing internal and/or external environments and circumstances.

Empowered living also includes the following:

- having the power to make decisions regarding your life
- having access to information and resources to help you make healthier and informed decisions
- having the ability to be assertive
- thinking positively regarding yourself and your situations
- having high self-efficacy and belief in your abilities to make change
- understanding the growth process and changes that are never ending and self-initiated
- increasing positive self-image and overcoming stigma,

In short, living empowered is the ability to function at the highest level of your consciousness to let go of self-defeating beliefs and behaviors and replace them with a high self-esteem, self-efficacy, and loving affirmations and positive behaviors.

## Con scious ness

Consciousness is innate self-awareness of one's personal identity, including the beliefs, attitudes, and behaviors. Consciousness also involves an awareness and understanding of how your beliefs, attitudes, and behaviors connect to and/or impact the world around you. Cultivating self-awareness is a preliminary action in beginning to accept and embrace yourself. Self-awareness empowers you to seek growth, which gives you the power to change and become who you really desire to be. When self-awareness becomes your reality, you do not feel the need to fit into others ideas of you nor do you feel the need to justify who you are and what you believe.

Empowered and consciousness go hand and hand. They are like two peas in a pod, working together to give you your foundation for growth and change.

Empowered consciousness is grounded in the belief that once you have self-awareness or "consciousness" of how negative beliefs, attitudes, and behaviors are obstacles to empowerment, then you are able to do something about it - make changes.

*Now the real work begins...*

*"Becoming intimately acquainted with your body, knowing the parts and how each part functions individual and together is one of the most important things you can do to protect it and pleasure it." — Dr. TaMara*

*"Have You Ever Stopped to Think about How Much Damage You've Done to Your Genitalia over the Years?"*

## CUTESY NAMES DON'T CUT IT!

Cunt, vajayjay, twat, slit, pussy, beaver, kitty, punanny, coota mama, coochie, black box, deep hole, down there, are just a few of the slang names that we use when referring to our genitalia. When you stop to think about it, many of these names are not cute at all! They are downright negative and derogatory. They send the wrong message about the female genitalia. Not only that, some of these words are very uncomfortable to hear. When we use these names and teach our girls to use cutesy names instead of using the correct terminology for body parts and functions, it takes away their value. When we devalue something, we do not respect it and take care of it. This lack of respect or value for our genitals places us at risk for sexually transmitted infections, HIV, and pregnancy and other intended and unintended consequences of sexuality because we do not value our body enough to protect it.

Using slang names also limit a girl and woman's ability to have an educated and informed conversation with their physician. Many physicians are not culturally competent. They do not understand the vernacular and slang names that are sometimes used when referring to body parts and functions. This lack of understanding can contribute to not receiving the necessary treatment and quality of care. The bottom line is that if the physician cannot understand you, then how can s/he help you?

Finally, because there are as many different slang names for each body part and sexual behavior as there are letters in the alphabet, it creates a communication barrier between parents and even our partners. So essentially, you could overhear your daughter having what appears to be an innocent conversation, but she really may be talking about sex! However, the unfortunate part about it is that you would not have a clue what she is saying because she is not using the correct terms. In addition, you may have missed the opportunity to intervene and/or provide her with the tools and skills to remain abstinence or negotiate safe sex.

Bottom line, we have to call it what it is! We use correct names for every other body part—we call an eye an eye or a leg a leg and not some other derogatory or degrading name. It is time to start calling a vulva a vulva and a vagina a vagina! Say it with me — out loud—VULVA, VAGINA! Anything less is wearing the stigma of shame that we have worn for so long!

## Activity: What's in a Name?

Materials Needed
Journal to write down terms and any personal reflections about this activity

Directions
Create a list of all the *slang terms* that you have used (or that you have heard) to describe the vulva and/or vagina. After you create the list, take a few moments to review and reflect on the terms.

Journal Questions to Consider

1. In what way(s) are these slang names associated with shame?

2. In what way(s) could these slang names be associated with risk?

3. How did this activity make me feel?

4. How did you feel reflecting on the slang names?

5. Did any particular names stand out more than others did? If so, please explain.

6. Do you use any particular names more than others? If so, which names?

7. After completing this activity, will you change any of the names that you use? If so, please explain. If not, please explain.

8. What did you learn from this activity?

## MOUND OF VENUS

*Carefully created to provide you pleasure*

*cultivating like a gardener I prune*

*shaving and trimming to perfection so smooth*

*you touch my mound of Venus*

*captivated by her beauty*

*suspended from her aura so breathtaking*

*you long to feel her so deep inside*

*you must,*

*experience her so surreal*

*into the Heavens…yes, she is miraculous*

*the power to give life*

*how extraordinaire*

*her pheromones drive you wild*

*in confidence she controls all*

*to her feminine wiles you so willingly submit*

*my mound of Venus*

*to it, be the glory!*

# CHAPTER 2:

# FEMALE REPRODUCTIVE SYSTEM

The female reproductive system is an amazing collection of organs that work together for the purpose of producing a new life and experiencing sexual pleasure. The reproductive system is among the most important systems in the entire body. Without the ability to experience sexual pleasure and reproduce, the human race would surely die off.

The female reproductive system, as amazing as it is, is very sensitive and prone to many health conditions such as sexually transmitted infections, infertility, cancers, and so much more. The reproductive health is influenced by many factors. These include age, lifestyle, habits, genetics, use of medicines, exposure to chemicals in the environment and so much more. Unfortunately, these influences may cause a woman to experience reproductive health challenges and quality of life issues such as infertility and sexual dysfunctions.

Reproductive health problems can be harmful to overall health, affect a woman's ability to get pregnant or sustain a healthy pregnancy, and impair a person's ability to enjoy a sexual relationship. Many problems of the reproductive system can be corrected with education, lifestyle changes, and/or proper treatment from a multidisciplinary team of care providers such as a gynecologist, obstetrician, sexologist, or sex therapist.

# IMPORTANCE OF KNOWING YOUR REPRODUCTIVE SYSTEM AND RESPECTING YOUR BODY

It is extremely important to become familiar with your reproductive system — after all, it is how we were created, and is an integral part of who we are! The reproductive system is just as important as all of the other systems in our bodies are. They are all interrelated and work together to provide optimal health.

It is so important that we touch our bodies and teach our girls that it is OK to touch their bodies too — after all, it is theirs. The more familiar we are with our body parts and how they function, the more we will be able to make healthier and informed decisions. Part of that learning includes properly taking care of our body and learning what is natural and healthy for our body. Not touching our bodies and/or teaching our girls not to touch their body only sends the message that their body parts and functions are something that is unnatural and nasty. It perpetuates the stigma and helps to create shame and guilt regarding their body. This negative view on their body will ultimately contribute to unhealthy ideals about sexuality.

The more familiar you are with your body parts and how they function, the more you will be able to make healthier and informed decisions. You will also be able to educate and empower your loved ones with the knowledges, skills, and tool they need to keep themselves safer. Not only that, you will be able to experience more intimacy and sexual pleasure. In addition, you will be able to communicate your beliefs, thoughts, wants, needs, and desires to your Beloved effectively.

Learning the proper terminology helps to remove language barriers and enables you to a have more informed conversation with your health care professional to get the care and treatment that you need. In addition, learning the proper terminology helps to add value to your body and when you value your body, you are less likely to place yourself at risk for STIs, unintended pregnancies and other emotional, mental, spiritual, social, legal, economical, chemical, energetical, political, institutional and physical consequences of sex.

After all, our bodies are a temple. If we do not take care of them, then who will? We only get one — there is no refund or exchange policy on our body, so we have to treat the only one we get with the utmost care and respect. At the end of the day, **you** are responsible for your sexual health. It is time to break the cycle and reclaim your sexuality! Knowing and understanding the value of your reproductive system and body is the first step to enhancing your sexual pleasure.

The female reproductive system includes the external genitalia and internal organs, which work closely together to help the system function properly and provide pleasure. The more you know about the reproductive system and how it functions, the better you able to provide yourself with pleasure.

Let us begin this fantastic journey into the female reproductive system. First up is the clitoris.

One of the most infamous, misunderstood, and under-appreciated organs is the **clitoris**, also known as the "pleasure spot." According to some researchers, stimulation of this organ accounts for 50 to 75 percent of most orgasms. Over 90 percent of women experience their first orgasm through its direct stimulation. Even more amazingly, most women experience multiple orgasms because of direct or indirect stimulation of this special spot of precious pleasure. With over 8,000 nerve endings — twice as many as the "mighty" male penis — it is no wonder why women can achieve multiple, mind-blowing orgasms.

So what exactly is she…the clitoris? Many women complain that their partner can't find her, mistreats her, or doesn't spend enough time getting to know her. The vast majority of women stimulate her in order to enhance their sexual experience! She is a key player to sexual pleasure. She is a small, round blossom of pinkish or brownish flesh located just above the vaginal opening. A true cutie, but shy at times! She's usually hiding under her custom designed hood, a soft fold of tissue called the "clitoral hood." It helps to protect it from over-stimulation. Her size and shape will differ from woman to woman, but on average, she is about two and a half to four inches long, similar to the length of a flaccid penis. (How about that?) However, it is important to note that her size does not correlate with the amount of pleasure she gives. Treat her right, give her the right stimulation and the results of magnificent multitude can be achieved no matter her length!

There's more to her than meets the eye! Only a small portion of her can be seen by the naked eye, since about 75 percent of her is hidden internally. Most people only focus on her pretty, bold head, or "glans." However, the clitoris is actually a complex network of nerves that stretch throughout the vagina and up into her woman's body. Some of her hidden internal parts include erectile tissue, glands, muscles, blood vessels, and nerves. Internal, Clitoris has a bulb winged-like figure that is reminiscent of a wishbone and sits on both sides of the urethra. These pretty wings are made of erectile tissue that extends beneath the inner lips of the vagina, and they fill with blood when her woman is aroused.

Once aroused, her bulb fills with blood, increasing her size and sensitivity, which may retract her hood to reveal her head. At the peak of pleasure or orgasm, she will return to her petite size. Sometimes when orgasm isn't achieved (or for some other reason), her bulb may remain full. If she remains full longer than a few hours, her condition and discomfort is pretty much the male equivalent of "blue balls.".

Next up is the **vulva**, which is home to the clitoris. The vulva is often times confused with the vagina — so, let's clear that up now. The vulva is the complete female genital package — the collective name for the external female genitalia located in the pubic region of the body. The vulva surrounds the external ends of the urethral opening and the introitus/opening of the vagina.

In addition to the clitoris, the vulva includes labia majora, labia minor, vulval vestibule, urinary meatus, and Bartholin's gland. The **vagina**, which I will explain in more detail later, is a passageway that connects your vulva with your cervix and uterus (womb) inside your body.

Affectionately referred to as "the lips," and literally translated as "large lips," the **labia majora** enclose and protect the other external reproductive organs. The labia majora are relatively large and fleshy, and are comparable to the scrotum in males. The labia majora contain sweat and oil-secreting glands. After puberty, the labia majora are covered with hair.

Just inside the labia majora, and surround the openings to the vagina and urethra lies the delicate folds of the **labia minora**. Literally translated as "small lips," the labia minora can be very small, or up to 2 inches wide.

The area between the labia minora is called the **vulval vestibule**, and it contains the vaginal opening and the urinary meatus. The **urinary meatus** is located below the clitoris and just in front of the vagina. The opening, or "**introitus**," of the vagina is located at the bottom of the vulval vestibule. The term introitus is more technically correct than "opening," since the vagina is usually collapsed, with the opening closed, unless something is inserted. The introitus is sometimes partly covered by a thin membrane called the **hymen**. Hymens are often different from person to person. Most women find their hymens have stretched or torn after their first sexual experience and/or vigorous activity such as horseback riding or exercise.

Located slightly behind, and to the left and right of, the opening of the vagina are the **Bartholin glands**. These two pea-sized glands secrete mucus to provide lubrication to the vagina when a woman is sexually aroused. The fluid helps slightly moisten the labial opening of the vagina to help make contact with this highly sensitive area more arousing and comfortable for the woman.

The internal reproductive organs in the female include ovaries, fallopian tubes, uterus, cervix, and vagina.

The **ovaries** are a pair of small glands about the size and shape of almonds, located on the left and right sides of the pelvic body cavity, lateral to the superior portion of the uterus. Ovaries produce female sex hormones such as estrogen and progesterone, as well as ova (commonly called "eggs"), the female gametes. Ova are produced from oocyte cells that slowly develop throughout a woman's early life and reach maturity after puberty. Each month during ovulation, a mature ovum is released. The ovum travels from the ovary to the fallopian tube, where it may be fertilized before reaching the uterus.

## PEARLS OF WISDOM

*During fetal life, there are about 6 million to 7 million eggs. From this time, no new eggs are produced. At birth, there are approximately 1 million eggs; and by the time of puberty, only about 300,000 remain. Of these, only 300 to 400 will mature to ovulation during a woman's reproductive lifetime. Fertility can drop as a woman ages due to decreasing number and quality of the remaining eggs.*

Attached to left and right top corners of the uterus and extending to the edge of the ovaries are a pair of muscular tubes called the **fallopian tubes**. The fallopian tubes end in a funnel-shaped structure called the **infundibulum**, which is covered with small finger-like projections called **fimbriae**. The fimbriae swipe over the outside of the ovaries to pick up released ova and carry them into the infundibulum for transport to the uterus. The inside of each fallopian tube is covered in cilia that work with the smooth muscle of the tube to carry the ovum to the uterus. **Conception**, the fertilization of an egg by a sperm, normally occurs in the fallopian tubes. The fertilized egg then moves to the uterus, where it implants into the lining of the uterine wall.

The **uterus**, also known as the womb, is a hollow, muscular, pear-shaped organ located behind and above the urinary bladder. It is connected to the two fallopian tubes on its top end and to the vagina (via the cervix) on its bottom end. The main function of the uterus is to support the developing fetus during pregnancy. The inner lining of the uterus, known as the **endometrium**, provides support to the embryo during early development. The visceral muscles of the uterus contract during childbirth to push the fetus through the cervix and the vagina.

The **cervix** is a cylinder-shaped neck of tissue that connects the vagina and uterus. The cervix is made of cartilage covered by smooth, moist tissue, and is about 1 inch across. Its name, cervix, comes from the Latin word meaning "neck" due to its role as the narrow connection between the larger body of the uterus above and the vagina below.

The cervix can be broken down into several anatomically distinct regions:

The **cervical canal** is the hollow orifice through the cervix that connects the uterine cavity to the hollow lumen of the vagina.

Connecting the cervical canal to the lumen of the vagina is a small, circular opening surrounded by the external tissue of the cervix also known as the **external os**.

Connecting the cervical canal to the uterine cavity is a small, circular opening where the cervical canal narrows before opening into the uterus, also known as the **internal os**.

The cervix produces cervical mucus that changes in consistency during the menstrual cycle to prevent or promote pregnancy. Lining the inside of the cervix is a thin layer of endometrium containing the epithelial cells that constantly produce cervical mucus. The cervical mucus that fills the cervical canal and forms a mucus plug blocking the flow of material between the uterus and the vagina. Around the time of ovulation, the consistency of the cervical mucus becomes much thinner, allowing the passage of sperm into the uterus for fertilization. The cervix plays vital roles in the control of movement into and out of the uterus, protection of the fetus during pregnancy, and the delivery of the fetus during childbirth. Additionally, during pregnancy the cervix and its mucus plug protect the developing fetus by sealing the uterus from possible contamination by external pathogens. During menstruation, the smooth muscle tissue in the myometrium of the cervix dilates to allow the passage of menstrual flow and may cause sensations of pain and discomfort known as menstrual cramps. Additionally, during sexual intercourse, the cervical mucus helps sperm move from the vagina through the cervix into the uterus.

Last, but certainly not least of the internal organs of the female reproductive system is the vagina. The **vagina** is an elastic, muscular tube that connects the cervix of the uterus to the exterior of the body. It is located inferior to the uterus and posterior to the urinary bladder. The vagina functions as the receptacle for the penis during sexual intercourse and carries sperm to the uterus. It also serves as the birth canal by stretching to allow delivery of the fetus during childbirth. During menstruation, the menstrual flow exits the body via the vagina.

**Q. I HAVE NOTICED CHANGES IN MY VAGINAL LUBRICATION. IS THIS NORMAL?**

A. The amount consistency, texture, taste, color, and odor can change depending on sexual arousal, the phase of the menstrual cycle, the presence of an infection, certain genetic factors, menopause, diet, etc. It is important to become intimately acquainted with your vagina's normal lubrication, so if there is a noticeable change in color (i.e. greenish yellow, grayish), consistency (i.e. clumpy white, too runny) and smell (fishy, foul), you can contact your physician to check for a presence of infection.

What would a conversation about the vagina be if I failed to mention the G-Spot? Very few issues in sexology, sexual medicine, and sex therapy instigate so much interest, debate, and controversy among clinicians and practitioners than the G-spot. One of the main reasons why the G-spot seems to garner much preoccupation and seems to be quite mysterious is because it seems as if not everybody can find it, nor is every woman able to orgasm through it.

The 17th-century Dutch physician Regnier de Graaf described female ejaculation and referred to an erogenous zone in the vagina that he linked with the male prostate; this zone was later reported by the German gynecologist Ernst Gräfenberg in the fifties. Beverly Whipple, a certified sex educator and counselor, and John D. Perry, an ordained minister, psychologist, and sexologist, named the G-spot after Ernst Gr Gräfenberg. Dr. Gräfenberg was the first modern physician to describe the area and argue for its importance in female sexual pleasure.

The "Gräfenberg Spot," more popularly known as the **G-spot**, is a spongy tissue that is located on the vagina's inner wall. When stimulated, this area of the vagina can lead to strong sexual arousal, powerful orgasms, and female ejaculation. This bean-shaped spot is reported to be located one to three inches up the anterior vaginal wall. It has also been reported that this highly sensitive area may be part of the female prostate. The key factor in finding the G-spot is becoming intimately acquainted with one's body. There are several things individuals can try to stimulate the G-spot. Because the G-spot is embedded in the muscle of the vaginal wall, it may require a little patience and effort to find. Every woman will respond differently; however, the more aroused the woman is the larger and more sensitive the G-spot becomes, making it easier to locate. The initial stimulation may cause a woman to feel a strong urge to urinate. However, this sensation passes after a short while and will be replaced by feelings of pleasure and arousal.


## CHANGES THAT HAPPEN IN THE VULVA OVER THE YEARS

### Fetus

As a fetus is developing, the appearance of the external genitalia is the same for both males and females during the eighth week. Around the third month of development, the external genitalia becomes defined. The genital tubercle becomes the clitoris. The urogenital folds become the *labia minora*, and the labioscrotal swellings become the *labia majora*.

## Childhood

At birth, a newborn girl's vulva may be swollen or enlarged as a result of having been exposed to the mother's increased levels of hormones. The clitoris is slightly enlarged. Once the mother's hormones wear off, both the vulva and clitoris with shrink in size. The vulva will not change much in appearance until puberty.

## Puberty

The onset of puberty produces a number of changes in the vulva and vagina—the vulva becomes larger, darkens in color, and may become more defined. Pubic hair begins to develop on the labia majora, later spreading to the mons pubis. The labia minora changes in appearance, becoming more prominent and darkened in color.

## Sexual arousal

Vulva tissue is highly vascularized, resulting in a number of physical changes in the vulva during sexual arousal. In response to sexual arousal, vaginal lubrication begins first, as the clitoris and labia minora increase in size and color. Increased vasocongestion causes the vagina to swell. The clitoris becomes erect and the glans become concealed by the clitoral hood. The labia minora increase considerably in thickness. Immediately prior to orgasm, the clitoris becomes engorged with blood, causing the glans to appear to retract into the clitoral hood. Rhythmic muscle contractions occur in the outer third of the vagina, as well as the uterus and anus causing an orgasm. An orgasm may have as few as one, or as many as 15 or more contractions depending on its intensity. Depending on the type of orgasm, it may or may not be accompanied by female ejaculation. During the plateau phase (explained later in the human sexual response cycle), the pooled blood begins to dissipate, the vagina and vaginal opening return to their normal relaxed state, and the rest of the vulva returns to its normal size, position and color.

---

<u>PEARLS OF WISDOM</u>
*Did you know that there is a difference between sexual arousal and sexual desire?* **Sexual arousal** *is a physiological response, whereas* **sexual desire** *is a psychological response. In other words, a woman can desire sex, but her body may not be prepared for intercourse, i.e. lacking vaginal lubrication OR a woman may not desire sex, but her body may be in an aroused state.*

## Childbirth

The vulvovaginal region may experience significant trauma during childbirth. During childbirth, the cervix, vagina, and vulva must stretch to accommodate the baby's head (approximately 9.5 cm (3.7 in)). This can result in tears in the vaginal opening and perineum. An episiotomy (the surgical cutting of the perineum) is sometimes performed to help facilitate delivery of the baby and to reduce the amount of tearing. The trauma caused to the vulva during childbirth will require a minimum of six weeks to heal properly and return to a state of normalcy.

## Menopause

During menopause, hormone levels decrease, and the body stops creating estrogen. Because of the loss of estrogen, the reproductive tissues that shrink in size, the vagina tends to become thinner, drier, and less flexible — a condition known as Vulvovaginal atrophy. Vaginal secretions are reduced, resulting in decreased lubrication. Reduced levels of estrogen also result in an increase in vaginal pH, which makes the vagina less acidic. Dwindling levels of estrogen levels reduces blood flow and moisture within the vagina, which can cause the vagina to shrink and tighten, creating higher risk for yeast infections and sexually transmitted infections. The mons pubis, labia, and clitoris are reduced in size.

## Activity: Becoming Intimately Acquainted

Materials Needed
Full-length floor mirror or hand held mirror and a journal to write down any personal reflections and about the activity.

Directions
*If using a full-length floor mirror:*

1. Sit on the floor facing the mirror.

2. Spread legs apart so that you are able to get a complete view your vulva.

3. Take a moment to notice the color, fullness, length, etc. of the labia majora (outside lips).

4. Using your fingers, gently explore the labia majora. Notice the texture, color, fullness, etc.

5. Using your fingers, gently spread the labia majora to view your labia minora.

6. Using your fingers, gently explore the labia minora. Notice the texture, color, fullness, etc.

*If using a hand held mirror:*

1. Prop the mirror up against the wall and follow steps 1- 6, or lie on the bed or the floor and follow steps 1- 6.

Journal questions to consider:
1. How did this activity make me feel?

2. What was my comfort level exploring my vulva?

3. Did I notice anything unusual about my vulva?

4. What did I learn from this activity?

# CHAPTER 3:

# FEMALE REPRODUCTIVE SYSTEM PHYSIOLOGY AND FUNCTION

The female reproductive system is designed to carry out several functions from intercourse, to pleasure, to create and bring forth life. All of the parts must work together in order for the system to function properly.

## THE MENSTRUAL CYCLE, PREGNANCY AND MENOPAUSE

### Oogenesis and Ovulation

Under the influence of **follicle stimulating hormone** (FSH), and **luteinizing hormone** (LH), the ovaries produce a mature ovum in a process known as **ovulation**. About 14 days into the reproductive cycle, an oocyte reaches maturity, and is released as an **ovum**. Although the ovaries begin to mature many oocytes each month, usually only one ovum per cycle is released. If an ovum is produced, but not fertilized and implanted in the uterine wall, the reproductive cycle resets itself through menstruation. The entire reproductive cycle takes about 28 days on average, but may be as short as 24 days or as long as 36 days.

### Menstruation

While the ovum matures and travels through the fallopian tube, the endometrium grows and develops in preparation for the embryo. If the ovum is not fertilized in time, or if it fails to implant into the endometrium, the arteries of the uterus constrict to cut off blood flow to the endometrium. The lack of blood flow causes cell death in the endometrium and the eventual shedding of tissue in a process known as **menstruation**. In a normal menstrual cycle, this shedding begins around day 28 and continues into the first few days of the new reproductive cycle.

The menstrual cycle is the monthly cycle of follicle and egg maturation, release of an egg (ovulation), and preparation of the uterine lining for pregnancy. If a woman does not become pregnant, the uterine lining tissue is shed as menstrual bleeding. Most menstrual cycles are 28 days in length. **Menarche** is the time in during adolescence when menstrual periods begin. Menstrual periods continue to occur until a woman reaches menopause.

Follicular phase. The **follicular phase** is the beginning of the menstrual cycle. It starts on the first day of the menstrual cycle and usually lasts about 14 days. The hormones follicle-stimulating hormone (FSH) and luteinizing hormone (LH) are released from the pituitary gland to stimulate the ovaries. In turn, the ovaries produce estrogen and stimulate the maturation of about 15 to 20 eggs in the ovaries inside small areas known as **follicles**. Once estrogen levels begin to rise, the secretion of FSH is reduced by a feedback system so that follicle stimulation ceases at the appropriate time. With time, one of the egg follicles (or rarely, two or more) becomes dominant, and maturation of the other follicles is interrupted. The dominant follicle continues to make estrogen.

**Ovulation** occurs at the midpoint of the menstrual cycle. Estrogen production from the dominant follicle leads to a sharp rise in LH secretion, causing the dominant follicle to release its egg. The egg is swept into the Fallopian tube by thin structures on the ends of the tubes known as fimbriae. At this time, the cervix produces an increased amount of thick mucus that assists sperm in the passage into the uterus.

Luteal phase. The **luteal phase** of the menstrual cycle begins at ovulation (egg release). After the egg is released, the empty follicle turns into a mass of cells called the **corpus luteum**. The corpus luteum then produces **progesterone**, a hormone that readies the lining of the uterus for implantation of a fertilized egg. If an egg has been fertilized, the fertilized egg travels down the Fallopian tubes back into the uterus and implants in the uterine lining tissue. If there has not been a fertilization of an egg, the lining of the uterus eventually is broken down and shed during menstrual bleeding.

**Q. IS IT SAFE TO HAVE SEX ON MY PERIOD?**
A. So you're "calling a code red" and closing up shop for maintenance because Mother Nature is calling about her "monthly evacuation?" Simply put, you are on your period and you are not feeling so frisky when "Aunt Flo's" in town. Well, you are not alone! Just the mere mention of the words sex and period in the same sentence, (and I don't mean the punctuation mark,) can make you feel totally grossed out and leave you cringing in disgust.

It is common for many women to avoid having sex while on their period. Just the thought of the blood, tampons, maxi pads, and fluctuation of hormones can totally ruin the mood. However, for some women, having sex while on their period is a natural part of life that comes with many benefits. It is also actually a turn on for many women because estrogen and testosterone start to rise by the third day of the menstrual cycle. Because of this spike in hormones, many women experience a heightened sense of arousal and feel an insatiable desire to be more sexual and sensual during this time. In addition, there are benefits to having sex during your menstrual cycle.

**Benefits? What benefits?**
Having sex during your period can potentially alleviate some of the discomfort of the menstrual cycle. The hormones and endorphins that the body releases during sex, such as oxytocin, helps to relieve mild pain, depression, and irritability associated with premenstrual syndrome (PMS). Having sex also increases blood flow, which has the potential to minimize headaches and relieve those dreadful cramps. If you are a little on the dry side, menstrual blood actually helps to keep the vagina lubricated, which will help to reduce uncomfortable vaginal dryness, ripping and tearing during intercourse. Additionally, with every orgasm, the muscle contractions helps to expel the blood flow and uterine lining much more quickly, thus making your period much shorter. Finally, many women enjoy sex more when they are on their period because of increased feelings of fullness in the pelvic and genitals. This feeling of fullness increases sensitivity and helps with arousal.

With all those benefits to having sex while on your period, why would someone choose not to partake in the pleasures of the period? Well, before you decide to get on your "surf board" and take a "ride the crimson wave," there are a few things to take into consideration:

Sexually Transmitted Infections (STI)
Practicing safer sex is even more essential during your period. Your risks of sexually transmitted diseases and infections are higher than normal during this time because the cervix expands more than usual to allow blood to flow. This expansion creates a direct pathway for bacteria and viruses to travel deep inside uterus and the pelvic cavity placing a woman at an increased risk for sexually transmitted infections. The vagina has a lower acidity at this

time, which puts the female at a greater risk of a yeast or bacterial infection, which also helps to aid in the transmission of STIs, hepatitis and other blood borne diseases. So on your period or not, safer sex is always the best bet.

It doesn't feel sexy!
Due to all the hormonal changes, cramping and bloating, you may not feel sexy or like being intimate during the "time of the month." You may feel unattractive or maybe your partner isn't comfortable with having sex during this time. These are very natural feelings. In order to move beyond this feeling, consider taking a hot and steamy shower with your Beloved. Not only will this help to relax you and spicy things up but it was also help to reduce any anxieties and concerns about cleanliness. Lots of foreplay will also help to take your mind off your period and onto your Beloved.

It can get messy!
Sex can be messy period, not pun intended. However, if you are concerned, here are a few ways to minimize the mess…

If you're worried about ruining your sheets, having sex on a towel will help to take those worries away and keep the sheets clean. You could also turn up your kink meter and consider investing in a pair of rubber sheets.

Having a warm, wet washcloth or wet wipes nearby to freshen up and for quick clean up afterwards can help to reduce the mess.

Your sex positions can also help lessen the mess. Having sex in the missionary position can limit blood flow. Try to avoid having sex in the female-on-top because there is the possibility of more leakage due to gravity.

Having sex toward the end of your period, when your flow is lighter will reduce the likelihood of coming in contact with a lot of blood.

Wearing a digraph, soft menstrual cup or a female condom can help reduce the amount of blood that might come out during intercourse. While these devices may not completely block menstrual flow, they can help absorb some of the blood and/or keep it off your partner.

If the mess really bothers you, try having sex in the shower. Since water can dry out the natural lubrication of the vagina, it might be a good idea to use a silicone-based lubricant also.

It's just nasty!
Men ejaculate. Women have vaginal fluid and periods. A period is nothing to fear. It is a totally natural, healthy biological process. Menstrual blood, like other bodily fluids, is natural. However, menstrual blood has been stigmatized and considered taboo by society. Historically, female bodies and feminine hygiene have been ostracized and made to feel dirty. Messages received by the media and feminine hygiene companies help to perpetuate this stereotype. In addition, some cultures and religions believe that a woman is unclean during her period. The decision to have sex on while on your period comes down to a personal choice that is based on your comfort level, beliefs, and values regarding sexuality and your partner's willingness to indulge.

I don't have to worry about getting pregnant, right?

Wrong! There is a chance that you can get pregnant while on your period. Although very rare and the likelihood of a woman getting pregnant is very low, it's still not **zero**. While every woman's menstrual cycle is different, in general women are usually most fertile about 14 days before the onset of their next menstrual period. This is called **ovulation**. You are likely to get pregnant if you have intercourse a few days before you ovulate, the day you ovulate, and a day or two after you ovulate. Depending on the regularity of their menstrual cycle, some periods last more than a week; some women may ovulate twice a month or even during their period. If you are not on a hormonal birth control method like the pill and are having unprotected sex during this time, there is a possibility of getting pregnant.

Period sex is not just intercourse—you have options!

If you and your Beloved have both moved beyond any hesitations about having sex while on your period, you're ready to take things to the next level. Instead of intercourse, allow your partner to earn their "Red Wings" through oral stimulation of the clitoris. To prevent your partner from coming in contact with any fluid that may be coming out of the vagina during this time, be sure to use a dental dam. If you do not have a dental dam, you can use a sheet of plastic wrap or cut a male condom in half and roll it out flat. Remember, oral sex carries the same risk as vaginal and anal sex, so make sure that you always practice safer sex.

Choosing to have sex during "that time of month" is a personal choice that both you and your Beloved have to make. Be informed and understand all the intended (and unintended) consequences of period sex. Make sure you have the conversation with your partner. Do not surprise your partner in the heat of the moment. Do not be misleading about what is going on with your vagina. Always be upfront and let them in on the decision prior to any sex play. Communication is the key to any sexual experience. As long as your partner is comfortable and you are practicing safer sex, there is no reason you can't enjoy sexual intimacy at all times, even during your menstrual cycle.

## Activity: Track Your Menstrual Cycle

Tracking your menstrual cycle simply means keeping a record of when you are menstruating and other information related to your cycle. Additionally, by tracking your menstrual cycle, you can get to know your body, learn what is natural for your body, and become an advocate for and authority on your own health. It can also help with family planning and pregnancy prevention.

Materials Needed
Menstrual Tracker and a journal to write down any personal reflections.

Directions:

- Download a menstrual tracker app to your phone, download a fillable menstrual tracker from an online website, or print out a menstrual tracker from an online website. You may also use an old-fashioned calendar.

- Using the menstrual tracker begin tracking your menstrual cycle. **Note the first day of your period.** The first day of your period is the day that you actually start to bleed. Your menstrual cycle runs from the first day of your period to the first day of your next period.

- Track your menstrual cycle for at least the next 21-35 days. Each woman or girl's cycle will be different.

- Keep track of any physical symptoms such as how many days you bleed, how many tampons or pads you use, cramps, breast tenderness, changes to vaginal fluids, or changes in appetite.

- Also, keep track of any emotional changes such as moodiness, feelings of anxiousness, crying spells, or irritability.

- Repeat each month.

<u>Journal questions to consider</u>:
1. How did this activity make me feel?

2. What did I learn from this activity?

3. Was this activity helpful in helping me to learn more about my menstrual cycle? If yes, please explain. If not, please explain.

4. How likely am I to continue using a menstrual tracker?

### Fertilization and Pregnancy

Once the mature ovum is released from the ovary, the fimbriae catch the egg and direct it down the fallopian tube to the uterus. It takes about a week for the ovum to travel to the uterus. If sperm are able to reach and penetrate the ovum, the ovum becomes a fertilized zygote containing a full complement of DNA. After a two-week period of rapid cell division known as the germinal period of development, the zygote forms an embryo. The embryo will then implant itself into the uterine wall and begin to form an amniotic cavity, umbilical cord, and placenta.

During the fetal stage, which lasts from 9 weeks after fertilization to birth, development continues as cells multiply, move, and change; the fetus grows larger and more complex until it is ready to be born. Pregnancy lasts an average of 280 days — about 9 months.

When the baby is ready to be born, its head presses on the cervix, which begins to relax and dilate. The mucus that has formed a plug in the cervix loosens, and with amniotic fluid, comes out through the vagina — that is known as "water breaking."

Once active labor begins, the walls of the uterus begin to contract. The contractions cause the cervix to widen and begin to open up enough for the baby to pass through. The baby is pushed out of the uterus, through the dilated cervix, and through the uterus/ birth canal. The baby's head usually crowns, or appears first; the umbilical cord comes out with the baby and is cut after the baby is delivered.

The last stage of the birth process involves the delivery of the placenta, which is now referred to as the afterbirth. After it has separated from the inner lining of the uterus, contractions of the uterus push it out, along with its membranes and fluids.

## Menopause

Menopause is defined as the absence of menstrual periods for 12 months. It is the time in a woman's life when the ovaries stop functioning causing the production of the hormones estrogen and progesterone to end. The process of menopause does not occur overnight, but rather is a gradual process called perimenopausal transition. There is no reliable lab test to predict when a woman will experience menopause. The transition into menopause is different for each woman. The average age of menopause is typically between 45 and 50 years of age, however menopause can occur as early as the 30s or as late as the 60s. Menopause can cause significant changes to the health and wellness of the vulva and vagina. I will address some of the changes in the following chapters.

# CHAPTER 4:

# THE PLEASURES OF THE FEMALE REPRODUCTIVE SYSTEM

The female reproductive system was created to experience pleasure—if not, then how is the clitoris explained? Remember, the clitoris is the only organ in the human body (both male and female) designed solely for pleasure!

## WHAT IS AN ORGASM?

An **orgasm** is a physical, emotional, mental, and spiritual response experienced at the height of sexual activity. Orgasm is also a biological release of chemicals and tension followed by pleasurable involuntary muscle contractions.

There are several types of orgasms a woman can experience: clitoral, vaginal, A-Spot G-spot, anal, full body, blended and multiple! I know you are probably thinking wait…women can have all those different types of orgasms? The answer is yes! Below is a description of the various types of orgasms:

### Clitoral Orgasm

The clitoris is the pleasure spot specially designed for women. It is the most sensitive area on the female body, and contains over 8,000 nerves. The vast majority of women experience clitoral orgasm through direct stimulation or indirect stimulation of the internal structure of the clitoris. Intensely pleasurable feelings start within the clitoris and send waves of pleasure throughout the body.

## Vaginal Orgasm

This kind of female orgasm begins deep in the vagina near the cervix and either stays focused in the pelvic and lower stomach areas. In fact, many women do not even realize that are experiencing a vagina orgasm because it begins so deep inside of the vagina. A vaginal orgasm may or may not happen in unison with a clitoral orgasm. During a vaginal orgasm, the uterus and pelvic muscles contract. The contractions are so strong that they can actually push anything that is inside of the vagina out, i.e., penis or sex toy. A vaginal orgasm takes longer to achieve. Continuous rhythmic thrusting is often the best way to bring a woman to a vaginal orgasm.

## A-Spot Orgasm (The Anterior Fornix Orgasm)

The A-Spot is located deep in the vagina, about 4-5 inches, on the front wall of the vagina. An A-Spot orgasm is achieved by stimulating this small patch of sensitive tissue, which is located near the cervix. When stimulated, the A-Spot can lead to rapid vaginal lubrication and arousal.

Also referred to as the *Epicentre*, this is a patch of sensitive tissue at the inner end of the vaginal tube between the cervix and the bladder, described technically as the 'female degenerated prostate.' (In other words, it is the female equivalent of the male prostate, just as the clitoris is the female equivalent of the male penis.) Direct stimulation of this spot can produce ferocious orgasmic contractions. Unlike the clitoris, it is not supposed to suffer from post-orgasmic over-sensitivity.

## G-Spot Orgasm

The G-Spot is located 2-3 inches inside the vagina on the front wall. The G-Spot is about the size of a nickel and the texture of the G-spot is much more spongy and coarse than the rest of the vagina. At first, it may be difficult for a woman to locate her G-Spot; however, it becomes much easier to find after she has had one orgasm. During sexual arousal, the tissue surrounding the urethra becomes engorged with blood and the Paraurethral/Skene's glands produce and fill fluid. The fullness of the gland stimulates the feeling of needed to urinate, partly because of the pressure of the fluids surrounding the glands of the urethra. Additionally, G-Spot orgasm is also responsible for the elusive female ejaculation.

**Anal Orgasm**

The Anus is an erogenous zone full of sensitive nerves. Additionally, the sphincter muscle creates intense sensations when it contracts. However, because the anus does not lubricate itself naturally, lots of lubrication — water-based or silicone-based — *must* be used during any anal play. There are several ways you can reach anal orgasm: manual stimulation; sex toy such as a vibrator, dildo, butt plug or anal beads; and/or oral-anal sex; or penile penetration.

**Cervical Orgasm**

The cervix is the entrance to the womb, the uterus. A woman's cervix is related to her feminine core, her sense of self, her heart, her creativity, and to her entire being. According to the Tantric tradition, a cervical orgasm is probably the most profound, meaningful orgasm a woman can experience. A cervical orgasm is characterized by contractions of the deep vaginal muscles and uterus. The sensation of cervical stimulation and orgasm feels different from clitoral stimulation, because they are responding to two different nerve-systems. A cervical orgasm will feel deeper, more intense and is accompanied by strong emotions, love, oneness with self, partner and god, ecstasy and transcendence, tears, crying and a feeling of deep satisfaction on all levels.

## Blended Orgasm

A blended orgasm is one of the most powerful orgasms a woman can experience. It offers a woman the best of both worlds. A blended orgasm is a potent combination of two or more types of orgasms occurring at the same time.

## Multiple Orgasms

Contrary to popular belief, multiple orgasms do exist, and they are entirely possible to achieve if there is little to no interruption in arousal or stimulation. Multiple orgasms come in quick succession, one after the other, usually with mere seconds to minutes between them. The challenge with multiple orgasms is that due to heightened sensitivity, continued orgasm may become uncomfortable if stimulation is continued. There are two types of multiple orgasms: sequential and serial. Sequential orgasms are orgasms that occur after one another with a few minutes in between. Additional stimulation is often required to get from one to the next, but there is no limit to how many you might have during one encounter. Serial orgasms are one orgasm experienced immediately after the next and the next and the next.

## Full Body/Expanded Orgasm

A full body/expanded orgasm is associated with Tantra. It can be describe as a true floating-on-cloud-nine outer body experience. A full body/expanded orgasm is the experience of feeling your whole body vibrating with orgasmic intensity and contractions that last from a few minutes to many hours.

These contractions and energetic sensations pulsate all over the body, especially in the abdomen, inner thighs, hands, feet, and genitals bringing about deep emotional release and rejuvenation, profound spiritual experiences, and an keen awareness not normally perceived in other types of orgasms. Full body/Expanded orgasm uses the body, mind, emotion, spirit, and sexual energy to create.

### Q. HOW DO I INCREASE MY CHANCES OF EXPERIENCING THE ULTIMATE ORGASM?

A. The quest to experience the ultimate orgasm is a challenge that many women will face throughout their lives. Below are some additional suggestions to enhance your orgasmic pleasure.

First, you may want to **consult with your physician** to rule out any medical condition that may be contributing to your inability to experience an orgasm.

**Mind play.** Keep in mind that sex begins in the brain. If there are any emotional or mental blocks during fore play and/or intercourse, then it will make it difficult to experience an orgasm.

**Know your body.** Always be aware of how you enjoy being touched sexually and you must communicate this openly and honestly with your partner. Share with him how you liked to be touched. Lovingly teach him and guide his hands all over your body.

Seduction is the key! Women need to be engaged in a lot of fore play prior to intercourse. **Set the mood. Don't just jump right into it.** Take your time and allow your intensity to build, as this will help to increase the intensity of your orgasm.

**Try different positions.** This allows for different types of stimulation of the vagina, G-spot, A-Spot and clitoris.

**Try using sex toys to bring yourself to orgasm.** There are a variety of sex toys on the market designed for specific usage. You may consider a clitoral vibrator or a g-spot vibrator to start you on your journey.

**Take your time.** Don't rush to the orgasm. Enjoy the full sexual experience, and slowly build up to your orgasm. If you can hold out, try to "edge" - control yourself just shy of the actual orgasm for as long as possible. The result of edging can be an extremely intense orgasm that will be accompanied with stronger contractions and a longer lasting climax.

**Strengthen your PC muscles.** Pubococcygeal muscles are a big part of the female orgasm. Try exercising your muscles using Ben Wa Balls, vaginal or Kegel Exercisers. The stronger the PC muscle the more intense the orgasm.

**Understand the Human Sexual Response Cycle.** Having an understanding of how your body responds during each phase of the human sexual response cycle will help to increase your chances of experiencing an orgasm.

**Stop having goal-oriented sex.** Don't focus so much on the goal but rather experiencing the sensuality and pleasure of your sex play.

**Delay the pleasure.** Women can delay orgasm through a variety of ways. For example, in some practices of Hinduism — such as Tantra, which emphasizes sexual intercourse for religious purposes — techniques allow some individuals to control ejaculation and orgasm.

When it comes to orgasms, it is important to note that orgasms vary in intensity, and women vary in the frequency of their orgasms and the amount of stimulation necessary to trigger an orgasm and even what type of orgasm she experience. Additionally, orgasms are affected by mental, emotional, social physical, spiritual, financial, environmental, medical, pharmacological, relational, etc. factors. So stop comparing your orgasmic experience to that of your girlfriends. No two orgasms are alike, not even your own. The important thing is to know your body, how it changes throughout the various stages of the Human Sexual Response Cycle, the different types of orgasms and orgasm techniques, increases the likelihood of having orgasms alone and/or with your partner.

*Pearls of Wisdom*
*Placing too much pressure on yourself to experience an orgasm can actually create shame. It is important to remember that having "goal-oriented" sex is actually counteractive. Relaxing into the experience will help to remove the pressure and the shame.*

## Self-Pleasure: Becoming Intimately Acquainted With Yourself

For many of people, masturbation or self-pleasure is a taboo topic. There are many harmful myths that exist about masturbation that may cause people to feel uncomfortable.

Society and the media does a great job at contributing to the taboo, stigma, and negative messages around sexuality. Marketing and advertising companies teach us that our bodies are dirty and disgusting. Constantly being inundated with such messages, beliefs, attitudes and feelings like these contribute to the unhealthy behaviors that put women at risk for HIV and other sexually transmitted infections, victimization, abuse, body image issues, unhealthy relationships, mental health challenges and so much more.

In some cultures and religions, masturbation is considered a sinful act. This can lead to guilt or shame about the behavior. Negative messages and feelings about masturbation can threaten our health and well-being. People who receive negative messages about masturbation when they are young often carry feelings of shame surrounding sexuality into adulthood, which can ultimately affect the way we interact in relationships and experience sexual pleasure.

In order to experience your sexuality fully, you have to move past the shame and peel back the negative and unhealthy layers of intergenerational patterns that surround sexuality. While masturbation was once thought of as a perversion and a sign of a mental problem, masturbation now is regarded as a natural, healthy sexual activity that is pleasurable and safe. According to various studies, masturbation is a very common behavior, even among people who have a sex partner. According to one national study, 95% of males and 89% of females reported that they have masturbated and here are some reasons why.

## The Clitoris connection!
Women have been perfectly designed with their own special pleasure spot! Did you know this spot is the only organ in the human body with the sole function of providing pleasure? In fact, most women usually experience their first clitoral orgasm through masturbation. When you know what you need to bring yourself pleasure and orgasm, you strengthen your connection to your body in addition to experiencing many other health benefits of masturbation.

## You learn more about your body
In order to experience pleasure, you have to be intimately acquainted with your body. Understanding your sexual response cycle and how your body changes during each cycle is the hallmark of sexual pleasure. Masturbation is a

great way to learn all about your body, your sexual response, and sexual triggers. Learning about what feels good to you can increase your chance of experiencing sexual pleasure with sex partners because it enables you to communicate your sexual turn-ons to your partners.

## Create an intimate bond

Some partners use mutual masturbation to discover techniques for a more satisfying sexual and intimate relationship. Through mutual masturbation, you learn about body mapping. This technique helps you learn what spots, various strokes, and techniques to use to please your partner and vice versa. In addition, mutual masturbation is a safer way to explore sexual activity with another person because it lowers your risk for unintended pregnancies, HIV, and other sexually transmitted infections.

## Increased confidence

There is a correlation between sexuality and confidence. Knowing how your body works, and what you are capable of helps to increase your confidence. The more confident you are the more likely you are able to make better decisions, creating stronger boundaries and facilitate healthier relationships. When you can bring yourself physical pleasure, you don't need someone else to that for you. Unsurprisingly, this knowledge leads to higher confidence and increased level of self-care that transcends beyond the bedroom.

*Added Health Benefits:*

Masturbation provides many health benefits that can help to enhance our physical, emotional, mental, and sexual health. Masturbation can:

- create a sense of well-being
- enhance partnered sexual experiences
- increase the ability to have orgasms
- improve relationship and sexual satisfaction
- improve sleep
- increase confidence self-esteem and improve body image
- provide sexual pleasure for people without partners
- provide treatment for some sexual dysfunctions
- reduce stress
- relieve sexual tension
- relieve menstrual cramps
- strengthen muscle tone in the pelvic and anal areas
- mutual masturbation can be a useful learning tool

Pleasuring oneself is one of the most powerful sexual experiences. The freedom to give yourself the permission to explore your body, the time, and space to feel pleasure, and to know that you are worth giving and receiving pleasure are some of the most powerful steps to becoming sexually empowered and liberated! Finally, in the words of Ru Paul, "if you can't love yourself, how in the hell are you going to love someone else?" If you do decide to show yourself a little love, trust me, you will not go blind!

At the end of the day, only you can decide what is healthy and right for you. If you feel ashamed or guilty about masturbating, consider talking with a sex therapist, educator, counselor, and/or clergy member to explore your beliefs and attitudes regarding sexuality.

## Activity: Bringing Myself Pleasure

Materials Needed
Journal to write down any personal reflections and about the activity. A sex toy such as a vibrator is optional.

Directions
1.  Prepare yourself for pleasure by setting the mood. Seduction is the key! Don't just take off your clothes and get right into it — relax and take your time. Entice yourself by performing a hot and sexy striptease. Start by turning on your favorite song to get you into the mood. Slowly begin peeling away all your clothes, layer by layer, until you are completely exposed.

2.  Take a relaxing bubble bath. Totally submerge your body in the hot and steamy water. Take deep breaths — inhale through the nose and exhale through the mouth. Massage your entire body as you lather with bubble bath or bath oil. Shave or trim up your private area. After about 30 minutes, dry off your entire body with a warm fluffy towel. Oil your entire body with your favorite body oil. Take your time to massage the oil into your skin.

3.  Use a mirror to explore your lady parts! Use a mirror to explore the outside of your anatomy. Familiarize yourself with all you behold. Admire and appreciate yourself just as you are. As you become more aware of yourself, you will be able to experience more pleasure.

4.  Slowly begin to pleasure yourself by tracing all of your curves and paying special attention to your sweetness. Gently caress your sweet spot using various strokes, motions, speeds, and pressure to enhance stimulations. Pay close attention to varying sensation as this will help you to be more in tune with your body as well as identify what turns you on. You

_Dr. TaMara Griffin_

may also considering using a vibrator to intensify the experience. Lubricant may also provide extra stimulation.

5. If you really want to heighten your experience, try completing steps in front of a full-length mirror. If you want to intensify your orgasm, pleasure yourself almost to the point of no return and just before you climax, stop. Doing this a few, times will help to increase your orgasmic intensity.

_Remember_:

No two vulva are alike! Just as women are created differently, so are vulvas. Each has its own distinct look. Lips vary in thickness, color, length, and shape. Just like anything else new, this may be weird or uncomfortable at first, but I encourage you to push through the feeling. If uncomfortable, repeat this exercise until you become more comfortable and intimately acquainted.

Journal questions to consider:

1. What were you taught about self-pleasure growing up?

2. How did this activity make me feel?

3. What are my current thoughts on self-pleasure?

4. What did I learn from this activity?

## SEXUAL CHOREOGRAPHY

Sex is a vital component of any relationship, and it is something most of us are not willing to live without. Sex drive, sex style, and sexual communication all weave together to create what I call "sexual choreography."

When's the last time you talked to your partner about your sex life together? Allow me to give you some talking points for each one of these complex elements of sexual choreography, so that you can develop a beautiful sexual dance with your beloved, and maximize your sexual compatibility.

### Sex Drive

Sexual desire and arousal are way more complicated than we think. Our sex drive is affected by a variety of things: hormones, life stressors, medical issues, environmental factors, relationship challenges, social factors, etc. Something as simple as a change in the weather can easily put a damper on the mood! Now add to that the uniqueness of you and your partner and here comes a whole new layer of complexities with each of your sexual thoughts, beliefs and behaviors. I strongly believe that differences in sex drive can be worked through as long as both parties are committed to putting in the required work.

Here are some talking points for you and your lover regarding sex drive:

- How often do you think we should have sex?
- How much sex is too much sex and/or when do you prefer sex?
- How do you perceive our balance of who initiates sex?
- What are your turn-ons and turnoffs?

- How important is foreplay to get you turned on?

It is also important to keep in mind that sexual desire and arousal, although closely linked, are two different things. Sexual desire is an emotional and mental response, while sexual arousal is the physiological response. So in essence, your partner may desire to have sex, but his or her body may not be responding physically. For example, her vagina may not be lubricating. Conversely, your partner may NOT desire to have sex, but their body may be responding. Keep that in mind and don't judge a situation if you don't know the facts.

**Sex Style**
Kinky, vanilla, freaky, romantic, bi-curious, hetero-flexible or a beautiful custom blend of a few — we all have a "sex style." Our sex style involves a combination of our learned thoughts and behaviors, favorite sexual positions, sexual preferences, and past experience but also includes our openness to different sexual experiences and experimenting. Our sex style can develop at any time and can also change, based on our growth and life experiences. Therefore, it is extremely important to learn how to be flexible – literally and figuratively! Allowing fluidity to exist in your sexual style increases your opportunities for experiencing pleasure. Of course, it goes without saying that all sexual experimentation with your sexual style should be safe, sane and consensual between adults.

Here are some talking points for you and your lover about sex style:
- Are you more traditional or open when it comes to sex?

- What positions do you enjoy?
- Would you consider yourself to be more vanilla or more kinky? What does that mean to you?
- Do you consider your sexual style to be fluid and flexible?
- Is your preferred sexual style monogamy or are you open to having sex with other people i.e. swinging, open relationships, threesomes?
- Do you like sex toys?
- Do you like rough sex or gentle sex?
- Do you like to switch up the routine?
- Do you like sex beyond the bedroom?

**Sexual Communication**

Your sexual frustration is your fault! Stop blaming your partner. We are responsible for our own sexual pleasure. We often set our partners up for failure because we think they should automatically know how to please, and this leaves us feeling frustrated. Teaching your Beloved might not sound sexy, but trust when you do, your sexual experience life will become a beautiful choreographed experience of synchronized movements, sounds and moments. To help choreograph your next "routine," perhaps you could consider taking a sexy and sensual sex education workshop together, play lover's games, try body mapping and guiding your lover's hand to your hot spots or just sit down and have a true heart-to-heart conversation, which brings me to my next point....Speak up!

Faked an orgasm? That's your fault! We have to learn to *speak up*! It is important that we communicate our sexual expectations, desires, beliefs, and attitudes to our partner, even if it feels unnatural in the beginning—just try! When we don't communicate, it sends the wrong message to our partners. When we don't talk with our partners and tell then exactly how we feel about our sexual experiences, we do them and ourselves a disservice. They may think they are pleasing us when they're not, and we are not receiving the pleasure we deserve. As a result, not only do we end up dissatisfied, we may end up resenting our partner, which may ultimately result in cheating. It is always important to remember that we are responsible for our sexual health and pleasure — that is we absolutely must communicate our wants, needs and desires.

Here are some talking points for you and your lover about sexual communication:

- Are you willing to talk about our sex life together?
- Have you ever faked an orgasm with me?
- Do you pretend to like techniques I use and secretly dislike them?
- Do you feel sexually satisfied with our sex life?

Our sexuality is not black and white. It exists on a spectrum of beautiful colors and complexities. Learning to understand the value and importance that each individual places on acknowledging, exploring and expressing their sexuality is key to creating sexual compatibility with our partners. Operating from this lens gives our partners the permission to fully express their sexual selves as well. This does not mean that you or your partner need to change fundamental parts of your sexuality, but rather choreograph your sex life together for ultimate sexual satisfaction.

# CHAPTER 5:

# THE PAINS OF THE FEMALE REPRODUCTIVE SYSTEM

## COMMON CONDITIONS OF THE FEMALE REPRODUCTIVE SYSTEM

A woman's reproductive system is the most fragile system in a woman's body. Given the extremely sensitive nature of the female reproductive system, women and girls are more vulnerable to disease and reproductive dysfunctions. According to The Center for Disease Control and Prevention (CDC), reproductive health problems are responsible for one third of health issues for women between the ages of 15 and 44 years. Nevertheless, sadly, many women are in the dark about pregnancy, ovulation, and female reproductive health. Reproductive health conditions include those that affect female external and internal organs along the reproductive tract. Some conditions may interfere with natural activity, while others may also affect reproductive functioning and fertility. Let's explore some of the common conditions that effect the female reproductive system.

### Infertility
Infertility is fairly common. Statistics show that about six percent women aged 15 to 44 years in the United States are unable to get pregnant after one year of trying. About twelve percent of women aged 15 to 44 years in the United States have difficulty carrying a pregnancy to term. Infertility is not

just a woman or girl's problem. Many couples struggle with infertility and seek help to become pregnant. Approximately ten to fifteen percent American couples are diagnosed with fertility problems. Infertility is defined as not being able to get pregnant after one year — or longer — of unprotected sex. Infertility may result from an issue with either you or your partner, or a combination of factors that interfere with pregnancy. For women, fertility relies on the ovaries releasing healthy eggs. Her reproductive tract must allow an egg to pass into her fallopian tubes and join with sperm for fertilization. The fertilized egg must travel to the uterus and implant in the lining. Infertility, however, does not always mean you are "sterile" — unable ever to have a child. Many women and couples who seek help can eventually have a child, either on their own, or with medical help.

The main symptom of infertility is not getting pregnant. Other symptoms may include irregular or absent menstrual periods. There may be no other obvious symptoms.

A number of factors may keep a woman or girl from getting pregnant:

- Polycystic ovary syndrome (PCOS). PCOS is a condition that causes women not to ovulate, or to ovulate irregularly. PCOS is the most common cause of female infertility.

- Damage to your fallopian tubes. The fallopian tubes be become damaged because of scarring from surgery, infections. If the fallopian tubes are damaged, the sperm cannot fertilize the ova (egg).

- Hormonal problems. The body may not be going through the usual hormone changes that lead to the release of an egg from the ovary and the thickening of the lining of the uterus.

- Cervical issues. Some women have a condition that prevents sperm from passing through the cervical canal.

- Uterine trouble. Polyps and fibroids that develop in the uterus can interfere with getting pregnant.

- Decline in the functioning of the ovaries. Ovarian reserves naturally decline with age resulting in a smaller about of healthy eggs. In addition, age menopause, medical reasons, surgery, perimenopause, or other health conditions may cause a decline in the ovaries functioning properly.

- Irregular menstrual cycles. Irregular menstrual cycles make it difficult for a woman to conceive because there is no predictable way to determine ovulation

- Untreated medical conditions. Untreated medical conditions, like chlamydia or gonorrhea can lead to pelvic inflammatory disease, which can cause infertility.

- Pelvic inflammatory disease (PID). Pelvic inflammatory disease is an infection of the organs of the female reproductive system. They include the uterus, ovaries, fallopian tubes, and cervix; all the organs a woman or girl needs to get pregnant and have a healthy baby.

- Genetics. Genetic factors such as chromosome abnormalities make it difficult for many women to conceive and/or deliver a healthy baby. Additionally, inherited genetic disease due to abnormal genes or mutations passed down from a parent can also cause infertility issues.

- Exposure to environmental toxics. Coming in contact with toxins in the air, food, water, buildings, soil and even common household products, can invade your body, affecting your organs and potentially causing fertility problems making in harder to conceive.

Risk Factors: Female fertility is known to decline with age; however, certain factors increase the risk of infertility in women and girls:

- age
- excessive alcohol usage
- excessive smoking
- one or more miscarriages
- extreme weight gain or weight loss.
- excessive mental, emotional and physical stress
- conditions of the female reproductive system i.e. PID, endometriosis, fibroids, etc.
- poor diet
- treatment for medical conditions

Infertility testing can be expensive, invasive, mentally and emotionally draining, and involve uncomfortable procedures. In addition, many medical plans may not reimburse the cost of fertility treatment.

The initial evaluation usually includes a tubal evaluation, and ovarian reserve testing and a semen analysis from the male partner. The physician will usually collect a medical and sexual history from both partners. He or she may also order a complete blood work up to check hormone levels, endometrial biopsy to examine the lining of the uterus, x-rays and/or laparoscopy to get a view of the female reproductive organs. Additional testing may include:

- Ovulation testing which measures the hormone levels in the blood to determine whether you are ovulating.

- Ovarian reserve testing which determines the quality and quantity of the eggs available for ovulation.

- Other hormone testing checks the levels of ovulatory hormones, as well as pituitary hormones that control reproductive processes.

- Imaging tests are used to see details inside the uterus that are not seen on a regular ultrasound.

- Genetic testing helps determine whether there is a genetic defect causing infertility.

Depending on what the physician learns during the initial testing, he or she will develop an individualized course of treatment. The physician will consider what is causing the infertility, how long you have been infertile, your age and your partner's age, as well as personal preferences. Options may include:

- Surgery to reconstruct reproductive organs or to remove polyps and fibroids

- Medications to help stimulate the ovaries and regulate ovulation

- Intrauterine insemination to help increase chances of fertilization by placing sperm in the uterus during ovulation

- Assisted reproductive therapy (ART) is when a woman's eggs are removed, mixed with sperm to make embryos that are placed back in the woman's body; it's successful about 11% to 39%, depending on the woman's age.

- In vitro fertilization (IVF) placed the already fertilized egg into the uterus. This is the most common ART

- ICSI (intracytoplasmic sperm injection): Sperm is injected directly into the egg in a dish and then placed into your uterus.

- GIFT (gamete intrafallopian tube transfer) and ZIFT (zygote intrafallopian transfer). Like IVF, these procedures involve retrieving an egg, combining it with sperm in a lab, and then transferring it back to the body. In ZIFT, the fertilized eggs are placed in the fallopian tubes within 24 hours. In GIFT, the sperm and eggs are mixed together before a physician inserts them.

- Egg donation involves removing eggs from the ovary of a donor who has taken fertility drugs. After in vitro fertilization, the fertilized eggs are implanted in the uterus.

- Assisted hatching assists the implantation of the embryo into the lining of the uterus by opening the outer covering of the embryo, which is referred to as hatching.

Most ART is done using the woman's own body. However, if there are severe problems, then the woman or couple may have to utilize a surrogate or gestational carrier.

**Surrogacy** involves the use of the woman's male partner sperm to fertilize another woman's egg. That woman carries the fetus to term. A **gestational carrier** is a woman who has an embryo (conceived by another couple) placed in her uterus, and carries the fetus to term.

There are several complications of infertility treatments. The most common complication of infertility treatment is a multiple pregnancy — twins, triplets or more. Generally, the greater the number of fetuses, the higher the risks, i.e., premature labor, premature delivery, or gestational diabetes. Fertility medications to induce ovulation can cause the ovaries become swollen and painful, abdominal pain, bloating and nausea. There is also a rare risk of bleeding or infection with assisted reproductive technology. Even with all the testing, treatments and counseling, there is no guarantee that you will get pregnant.

Infertility can take a toll on a woman's mental, emotional, physical, spiritual, social, biochemical, financial, legal, institutional well-being. If you or a woman you know is experience issues with fertility, please consider a multidisciplinary approach including but not limited to gynecologist, reproductive endocrinologist, infertility specialist, embryologist, sex therapist or counselor to work together in order to achieve success.


**Dyspareunia**

Dyspareunia is recurrent or persistent genital pain before, during, or after sex. It can be acquired, congenital, generalized, or situational. Dyspareunia is not a disease, but rather a symptom of an underlying physical, biological, or psychological factor. The pain, which is often described as excruciating menstrual cramps, can be mild or severe. It may be superficial, felt in the area around the opening of the vagina and vulva.

Dyspareunia is a condition that has many causes and is not a diagnosis of itself. Some of the causes for dyspareunia may include vaginismus (a condition that affects a woman's ability to tolerate vaginal penetration), insufficient vaginal lubrication, vaginal thinning, and dryness of the vaginal wall. Medical conditions such as endometriosis, cancer, ovarian cysts, fibroid tumors, sexually transmitted infections, and pain from bladder irritation can also cause dyspareunia. An injury to the genital area or past surgeries that have left scar tissue sometimes result in vaginal pain, along with inadequate foreplay and certain sexual positions.

Some symptoms of dyspareunia may include a burning, ripping, tearing, or aching feeling associated with vaginal penetration. The pain may also be felt throughout the entire pelvic area and the sexual organs, especially during deep thrusting or with certain sexual positions.

Determining whether the pain is more superficial or deep is important in understanding what may be causing pain and provide options for more effective treatment. Depending on the root cause, treatment options include estrogen therapy, sex therapy, and medication. Because symptoms of dyspareunia may mimic symptoms of other reproductive health conditions, including sexually transmitted infections, it is extremely important that you speak with your physician and/or sex therapist about your concerns. DO NOT try to diagnose yourself!

### Endometriosis

Endometriosis is estimated to affect over one million women and girls, ages 16 and 50, in the United States. Many women with endometriosis will experience pain just before, during, or after menstruation is the most common symptom. Some women and girls will also experience during or after sex, or during bowel movements or urination. Others report experiencing ongoing pain in the pelvis and lower back, fatigue, infertility and other gastrointestinal upsets such as diarrhea, constipation, and nausea. Some women with endometriosis have no symptoms at all. The severity and frequency of symptoms may be related to the location of the growths.

Complications of endometriosis include internal scarring, adhesions, pelvic cysts, chocolate cyst of ovaries, ruptured cysts, and bowel and ureteral obstruction resulting from pelvic adhesions. Endometriosis-associated infertility can be related to scar formation and anatomical distortions due to the endometriosis.

Although the exact cause of endometriosis is not certain, several possible explanations include:

- **Retrograde menstruation.** This is the most likely explanation for endometriosis. In retrograde menstruation, menstrual blood containing endometrial cells flows back through the fallopian tubes and into the pelvic cavity instead of out of the body. These displaced endometrial cells stick to the pelvic walls and surfaces of pelvic organs, where they grow and continue to thicken and bleed over the course of each menstrual cycle.

- **Embryonic cell growth.** The cells lining the abdominal and pelvic cavities come from embryonic cells. When one or more small areas of the abdominal lining turn into endometrial tissue, endometriosis can develop.

- **Surgical scar implantation.** After a surgery, such as a hysterectomy or C-section, endometrial cells may attach to a surgical incision.

- **Immune system disorder.** A problem with the immune system may make the body unable to recognize and destroy endometrial tissue that is growing outside the uterus.

There is no definite way to determine who will have endometriosis, but research shows that the condition is more common in women who:

- are in their 30s and 40s
- have not had children
- have periods longer than seven days
- have cycles shorter than 28 days
- started their period before age 12
- have a mother or sister who had endometriosis

To diagnose endometriosis, a physician will check the ovaries, uterus, and cervix for anything unusual. An exam can sometimes reveal an ovarian cyst or internal scarring that may be due to endometriosis. He or she may also do a pelvic exam, ultrasound, or laparoscopy.

Treatment for endometriosis is usually with medications or surgery. Depending on the severity of symptoms (and whether or not you hope to become pregnant), the physician may offer the following options: pain medication, hormone therapy, hysterectomy. Alternative therapy includes acupuncture.

### Vaginismus

Vaginismus is the physical or psychological condition that affects a woman or girl's ability to tolerate in vaginal penetration because of involuntary vaginal muscle spasms.

A woman or girl suffering from vaginismus cannot consciously control the spasm. The involuntary muscle spasm makes penetration painful or impossible, as the reflex happens because of an object such as a penis, vibrator, tampon, etc. coming towards it. In some cases, even the thought of the object can cause the vagina to spasm.

Vaginismus can be either primary or secondary. A woman or girl diagnosed with **primary vaginismus** has never been able to have penetrative sex or experience vaginal penetration without pain. **Secondary vaginismus** occurs when a woman who has previously been able to achieve penetration develops vaginismus.

The exact cause of vaginismus is unknown; however, it may be due to physical causes such as an infection or trauma. Some cases of vaginismus may be due to psychological causes like fear or anxiety. Other factors that contribute to vaginismus may include:

- medical conditions such as pelvic inflammatory disease, ovarian cysts, endometriosis, cancer, urinary tract disorders, etc.
- psychophysiological reaction to sexual intercourse based on a negative past experience
- sexual trauma
- scarring
- vaginal thinning and dryness
- incomplete sexual arousal
- low estrogen
- inadequate foreplay
- sexually transmitted infections

- allergies to spermicides or latex condoms
- not trusting one's partner
- body image issues
- misconceptions about sex
- conservative family upbringing
- first time sex anxiety

Symptoms of vaginismus include a burning, ripping, tearing, or aching sensation associated with penetration. The pain can be at the vaginal opening, deep in the pelvis, or anywhere between. Pain may also be felt throughout the entire pelvic area and the sexual organs and may occur only with deep thrusting.

The treatment for vaginismus is aimed at identifying and properly treating the underlying disorder. For example, medications are usually prescribed to treat any infections. Water-based or silicone-based lubricant may be recommend to help ease vaginal friction and discomfort during intercourse. Vaginal dilation exercises may be used to treat vaginismus. Vaginal dilation therapy should only be done under the direction of a physician or sex therapist. Sex therapy can also be used to address underlying psychological causes of vaginismus. Sex therapy can provide tools, techniques, and educational resources.

The treatment for secondary vaginismus is the same as for primary vaginismus, although, in these cases, previous experience with successful penetration can assist in a more rapid resolution of the condition.

Each case of vaginismus is different. An individualized comprehensive integrative approach to treatment is the most effective. The condition can be manageable if you are proactive and stay on top of your health. Work with your physician and/or sex therapist to get treatment, learn what works best for you.

## Lichen Sclerosus

Lichen Sclerosus is a long-term problem of the skin. It mostly affects the genital and anal areas. Lichen Sclerosus is a skin condition only and does not extend into the vagina or inside the anus. Sometimes, Lichen Sclerosus appears on the upper body, breasts, and upper arms. Lichen Sclerosus is most commonly seen in post-menopausal women. Lichen Sclerosus can make sex (and even urination) extremely painful due to itching and scarring. Scarring may narrow the opening of the vagina, which can make penetration painfully difficult. In addition, blistering of the skin may make the vulva unbearable to touch. If a young girl gets lichen sclerosis, she may not require lifelong treatment. Lichen Sclerosus sometimes goes away at puberty.

The exact cause of lichen sclerosis is unknown. However, but may be the result of an overactive immune system and hormone problems. Although Lichen Sclerosus may involve the skin around the genitals, it is not contagious and cannot be spread through sex.

Symptoms of Lichen Sclerosus include small white, shiny, smooth spots on the skin that grow into bigger spots overtime becoming thin and crinkled. If the disease is a mild case, there may be no symptoms. Other symptoms of Lichen Sclerosus are:

- itching (very common)
- discomfort or pain
- bleeding
- blisters

In the case of severe lichen Sclerosus, a physician can identify the condition by observation; however, he or she will do a biopsy to confirm diagnosis. If Lichen Sclerosus is diagnosed it is usual also to do a routine blood test to check for an underactive thyroid gland. This is because of the association between Lichen Sclerosus and autoimmune diseases.

Lichen Sclerosus of the genital skin should be treated. Even if it isn't painful or itchy, the patches can scar. This can cause problems with urination or sex. Unfortunately, there is no cure for lichen Sclerosus. Typical treatment for Lichen Sclerosus involves topical prescription-strength steroid cream or ointment. Surgery is normally not a good option for women. When the Lichen Sclerosus patches are removed from the genitals of women and girls, they usually come back. Treatment does not fix the scarring that may have already occurred.

Lichen sclerosis can create shaming issues such as feelings of isolation, hopelessness, low self-image, depression, anxiety, anger and so much more. Some women and girls may suffer from low self-esteem and sex-esteem. Sex therapy, counseling, and education, in addition to medical treatment, should also be concerned as an additional effective treatment option.


## Vaginal Atrophy

Vaginal atrophy, (also called atrophic vaginitis or vulvovaginal atrophy) is an inflammation of the labia, vagina, opening of the vagina and the outer urinary tract. This inflammation is likely due to a lack of the reproductive hormone estrogen. The lack of estrogen causes thinning, drying and lack of lubrication of the vaginal walls.

Vaginal atrophy can occur at any time in a woman's life; however, the most common cause of vaginal atrophy is the natural decrease in estrogen that happens during menopause. However vaginal atrophy condition can occur as a result of other conditions that decrease estrogen in the body such as: decreased ovarian functioning due to radiation therapy or chemotherapy, immune disorder, removal of the ovaries, entering the post-partum period, and lactation. Various medications can also cause or contribute to vaginal atrophy. The more estrogen levels fall, the more severe the symptoms of vagina atrophy may become.

The initial symptom is often lack of lubrication during intercourse. Eventually, persistent vaginal dryness may occur. Additional symptoms of vaginal atrophy can include vaginal itching, soreness and itching, as well as painful intercourse, and bleeding after sexual intercourse and/or white discharge, malodorous discharge due to infection. The shrinkage of the tissues and loss of flexibility can be extreme enough to make intercourse impossible. For many, vaginal atrophy can also lead to agonizing urinary symptoms. Given the interconnected of the vaginal and urinary symptoms of this condition is sometimes referred to genitourinary syndrome of menopause (GSM). Urinary symptoms include painful urination, blood in the urine, increased frequency of urination, incontinence, and increased likelihood and occurrence of infections. The symptoms of GSM may begin during perimenopause. As estrogen levels begin to fall, you may begin experiencing early signs of GSM. As the estrogen levels fall more dramatically, symptoms may become more severe.

Given that menopause is a natural progression of the female reproductive system - sometimes based on health conditions, some women will experience an early menopause - most women will experience varying degrees of vagina atrophy. However many women do not actively seek out treatment because of shame, self-treatment, and/or they feel that the symptoms are not significant enough to report. Diagnosis of vaginal atrophy and GSM includes a pelvic exam, urine exam, and acid balance test. Early treatment options may not be enough for relief. Treatment during later periods of menopause may focus on boosting estrogen levels to decrease discomfort and symptoms. Treatment may include vaginally administered estrogens. Additionally, the use of water-based lubricants and regular sexual activity can be helpful. Before beginning any treatment, it is important to consult with your physician to determine the right treatment for you.

There is no definitive way to prevent vagina atrophy and GSM, but you may be able to reduce your risk. Regular sexual activity may help boost your overall vaginal health. The increased blood flow can help keep your vaginal tissues healthy. Finally, try to avoid anything that may lower the natural estrogen levels in your body.

## Uterine Fibroids

It is estimated that sometime during their childbearing years between twenty and fifty percent of women of reproductive age have fibroids, although not all are diagnosed. Fibroids range in size from range in size, from the size of a pea to the size of a small grapefruit. Only about one-third of these fibroids are large enough to be detected by a health care provider during a physical examination.

Uterine fibroid tumors are muscular growths that form a fibrous "knot" or "mass" within the wall uterus. Uterine fibroids are noncancerous growths of the uterus that often appear during childbearing years. Uterine fibroids are not usually associated with uterine cancer; however, rarely (less than one in 1,000) a cancerous fibroid will occur.

There are four types of fibroids. They are categorized based on their location:

- **Intramural fibroids.** Intramural fibroids are the most common type of fibroid. These fibroids are normally found in the wall of the uterus. Intramural fibroids may grow larger and can stretch your uterus.

- **Submucosal fibroids.** These types of tumors develop in the middle muscle layer (myometrium) of your uterus. Submucosal tumors are not as common as other types, but when they do develop, they may cause heavy menstrual bleeding and trouble conceiving.

- **Subserosal fibroids.** Subserosal fibroids form on the outside of your uterus, which is called the serosa.

They may grow large enough to make your womb appear bigger on one side.

- **Pedunculated Fibroids.** When Subserosal or submucosal fibroids develop a stem, they become pedunculated fibroids. Pedunculated fibroids can grow out from the surface of the uterus or into the cavity of the uterus.

The exact cause of fibroids remains unclear. However, researchers believe that the combination of hormones effected by estrogen and progesterone and family history could play a role. Race may also appears to play a role. Black women are two to three times more likely to develop fibroids than women of other races are. Black women also tend to develop fibroids at a younger age and may have symptoms from fibroids in their twenties, whereas White women tend to develop symptoms during the thirties and forties. Adolescent girls may rarely develop fibroids. Onset of menses prior to age ten may increase the risk.

Many women who develop fibroids may not experience any symptoms. However when symptoms are present, they can become extremely painful and debilitating. Fibroids can cause a number of symptoms depending on their size, location within the uterus, and how close they are to adjacent pelvic organs. Abnormal uterine bleeding, pain, and pressure are the most common symptoms. Symptoms may manifest as:

- heavy or prolonged menstrual periods
- bleeding between menstrual periods
- pelvic pain
- frequent urination

- low back pain
- pain during intercourse
- iron-deficiency anemia

Each woman may experience symptoms differently, therefore it is extremely important to pay close attention to your body and take note of any changes.

Fibroids are most often found during a routine pelvic examination. If a fibroid is suspected, the physician will order additional testing such as an ultrasound to help confirm diagnosis and differentiate it from other conditions such as ovarian tumor. When trying to determine if a fibroid is present in the uterine cavity, a hysterosonogram is performed. Magnetic Resonance Imaging (MRI) and Computed Tomography (CT) scans can also play a role in diagnosing fibroids. In the case of heavy abnormal bleeding, the physician may also order a blood test to check for iron-deficient anemia.

Treatment for fibroids usually depends on the combination of symptoms, the location of the fibroid, the number, the size, the woman's age and childbearing potential. In addition, since most fibroids stop growing or may even shrink as a woman approaches menopause, the physician may suggest an observation before moving forward with treatment. **Options for the treatment of uterine fibroids include surgery and medication management:**

- **Hysterectomy** involves the surgical removal of the uterus and sometimes the cervix, fallopian tubes and ovaries. Fibroids remain the number one reason for hysterectomies in the United States.

- **Myomectomy** involves removing the fibroids, but leaving the uterus intact to enable a future pregnancy.

- **Gonadotropin-releasing hormone agonists (GnRH agonists)** lowers the level of estrogen creating a pseudo menopause. This helps to shrink the fibroid making surgical treatment easier.

- **Uterine artery embolization (UAE).** Uterine artery embolization is a newer, minimally invasive technique that is used to embolize, or cut off, the arteries supplying the blood to the fibroids. By cutting off the blood flow, the fibroids shrink in size.

For the most part, fibroids that do not cause a problem for the woman can be left untreated. However, the risk of leaving these fibroids in place is that they sometimes grow to a size that eventually cause significant symptoms, thus requiring removal.

### Q. CAN I STILL GET PREGNANT IF I HAVE FIBROIDS?

A. The good news is that you can still get pregnant and a have normal pregnancy. The difficult news is that you may experience some complications. The size of the fibroid and its precise location within the uterus are all-important factors in determining whether a fibroid causes complications. Research suggests that certain types of uterine fibroids can change the size and shape of the uterus, affecting a woman's ability to get pregnant. Fibroids are also linked to a greater risk of cesarean delivery and a risk of heavier bleeding after delivery. If you are trying to get pregnant, talk with your obstetrician for care regarding your specific situation.

**Gynecologic Cancers**

Every six minutes, a woman in America is diagnosed with gynecologic cancer. According to the American Cancer Society, about 90,000 women in the United States are diagnosed annually with cancers affecting the reproductive organs; nearly one-third will lose their lives. Some of these gynecologic cancers have been called "silent killers" because women are often unaware of the signs and symptoms associated with these cancers and do not catch them until it is too late.

### WHAT ARE GYNECOLOGIC CANCERS?

Gynecologic cancer is an uncontrolled growth and spread of abnormal cells that originate from the reproductive organs. These cancers can occur in any part of the female reproductive system.

The most common reproductive cancers in women are uterine (endometrial), cervical, ovarian, vaginal and vulvar.

### UTERINE CANCER

Uterine cancer, also known as endometrial cancer, is the most common type of gynecologic cancer. Each year, approximately 50,600 women in the United States get uterine cancer. It is the fourth most common cancer in women in the United States and it is the most commonly diagnosed gynecologic cancer. There are two main types of uterine cancer: Endometrial and uterine sarcoma. Endometrial cancer is the most common and it affects the endometrium — the lining of the uterus. Uterine sarcoma is a rare form of uterine cancer that forms in the muscle and tissue that support the uterus. Uterine cancer usually occurs in women age 55 or older, however younger women are still susceptible to getting this type of cancer.

## CERVICAL CANCER

Cervical cancer is the second most common cause of death by cancer in women. In the United States alone, 12,000 women are diagnosed with cervical cancer each year and about 4,000 die from it. Most cervical cancers (80 to 90 percent) are squamous cell cancers. Adenocarcinoma is the second most common type of cervical cancer, accounting for the remaining 10 to 20 percent of cases. Almost all cervical cancers are caused by Human Papillomavirus (HPV). A woman or girl can get HPV by having sexual contact with someone who has a cancer causing strain of the virus. A woman or girl with a persistent HPV infection is at greater risk of developing cervical cell abnormalities and cancer. Cervical cancer is also more likely in women or girls who smoke, have HIV or AIDS, have poor nutrition, and who do not get regular Pap tests. Cancer of the cervix tends to occur during midlife. Although half of the women diagnosed with the disease are between 35 and 55 years of age, younger women are still susceptible to getting this type of cancer.

## OVARIAN CANCER

Ovarian is the eighth most common cancer among women in the United States, excluding non-melanoma skin cancers. However, it is the fifth most common cause of cancer deaths in women. Among the gynecologic cancers (uterine, cervical, and ovarian), ovarian cancer has the highest rate of deaths - five (5) year survival rate if diagnoses is made early before. There are three types of ovarian cancer. The type of cell where the cancer begins determines the type of ovarian cancer you have. The ovarian cancer types include epithelial, germ cell, and stromal cell cancer. Epithelial ovarian cancer is the most common, accounting for 85 to 89 percent of ovarian cancers. About seven percent are stromal. Germ cell is rare for of ovarian cancer that tends to occur in younger girls. Ovarian cancer is more likely to occur as women get older however, younger women are still susceptible to getting this type of cancer.

### VAGINAL CANCER

Vaginal cancer is one of the rarest forms of gynecologic cancers, usually affecting women between 50 to 70-years-old. About 2,000 women are affected by vaginal cancer in the United States each year. According to the Centers for Disease Control and Prevention (CDC), 75 percent of vaginal cancers are associated with HPV. Black and Hispanic women more commonly get HPV-related vaginal cancer than women of any other race or ethnicities. There are four types of vaginal cancer: squamous cell carcinoma, adenocarcinoma, clear cell adenocarcinoma and melanoma. Squamous cell carcinoma makes up 85% to 90% of vaginal cancers. It develops slowly through a precancerous condition called vaginal intraepithelial neoplasia. Adenocarcinoma begins in the vaginal gland tissue. It makes up about 5% to 10% of vaginal cancers. Clear cell adenocarcinoma is a rare Adenocarcinoma. This cancer occurs in women whose mothers took the drug diethylstilbestrol (DES) during pregnancy between the late 1940s and 1971. Melanoma is extremely rare malignancy that is associated with high risk of recurrence.

### VULVAR CANCER

Vulvar cancer is a rare type of cancer. It forms in a woman's external genitals, called the vulva. Vulvar cancer most often affects the labia majora. Less often, cancer affects the labia minora, clitoris, or vaginal glands. It is estimated that about 4,490 cases of vulvar cancer will be diagnosed. Vulvar cancer usually forms slowly over a number of years.

Vulvar cancer is named for the type of tissue where the cancer started. The most common type of vulva cancer is squamous cell carcinoma. **Squamous cell carcinoma is a type of skin cancer that accounts for about 90 percent of vulvar cancers, most of which are found on the labia.**

Squamous cancer can develop through a "precancerous" condition, called vulva intraepithelial neoplasia (VIN). VIN is a premalignant growth of cells on the vulva and is treated differently from invasive cancer.

There are several subtypes of squamous cell carcinoma:

- The **keratinizing type** is most common subtype and it usually develops in older women. This subtype is not linked to infection with human papilloma virus (HPV).

- **Basaloid** is less common subtype and is more often found in younger women with HPV infections.

- **Verrucous carcinoma** is another uncommon subtype that is slow grow.

Other less common types of vulvar cancer include adenocarcinoma, melanoma, and Sarcoma. These cancers account for approximately 10 percent of vulvar cancers.

**Adenocarcinomas**. Vulvar adenocarcinomas is found on the sides of the vaginal opening. It most often start in cells of the Bartholin glands. Every eight out of 100 women with get this type of vulvar cancer. Cancer can also form in the sweat glands of the vulvar skin. Paget's disease of the vulva is a condition in which adenocarcinoma cells are found in the top layer of the vulvar skin. Up to 25% of patients with vulvar Paget's disease also have an invasive vulvar adenocarcinoma.

**Melanoma**. Vulvar melanomas are rare, accounting for about 2% to 4% of vulvar cancers. It occurs most often on the clitoris or the labia minora. Women with melanoma on other parts of their body have an increased risk of developing vulvar melanoma.

**Sarcoma**. Less than two of every 100 vulvar cancers are sarcomas. Unlike other cancers of the vulva, vulvar sarcomas can occur in females at any age, including in childhood.

Vulvar cancer most often affects women 65 to 75 years of age. However, it can also occur in women 40 years of age or younger.

Unfortunately, most women are not aware of the signs and symptoms of gynecological cancers. In addition, many of the symptoms that are related to gynecological cancers are very similar to symptoms of other female reproductive health conditions. One way to recognizing when a common symptom might actually indicate cancer is for women to becoming intimately acquainted with their body and to know what is natural for their body.

Learning the signs and symptoms of gynecological cancers can help result in early detection and treatment. Signs and symptoms are not the same for everyone and each gynecologic cancer has its own signs and symptoms. See the chart on the next page for signs and symptoms of gynecological cancers.

| Symptoms | Cervical Cancer | Ovarian Cancer | Uterine Cancer | Vaginal Cancer | Vulvar Cancer |
|---|---|---|---|---|---|
| Abnormal vaginal bleeding or discharge | ● | ● | ● | ● | |
| Feel full too quickly or difficulty eating | | ● | | | |
| Pelvic Pain or pressure | | ● | ● | | |
| Frequent or urgent need to urinate and/or constipation | | ● | | ● | |
| Bloating | | ● | | | |
| Abdominal or back pain | | ● | | | |
| Itching, bringing, pain, or tenderness of the vulva | | | | | ● |
| Changes in vulva color or skin such as a rash, sores, or warts | | | | | ● |

Although many of the symptoms associated with gynecologic cancers discussed may seem common and often times are due to other causes, it is important to pay attention to any changes. If you notice new symptoms that are occurring almost daily for more than a few weeks this can be a sign that you need to go see a physician.

Of course, there is no guaranteed way to know for sure if a woman or girl will get a gynecologic cancer but knowing the signs and symptoms, getting regular examines and screenings, maintaining healthy lifestyle and behavior choices, knowing your family history will definitely help you to be proactive in reducing your risk and/or early detection.

Even still, every woman is at risk for developing a gynecologic cancer. It is important to learn what types of cancers there are and know their signs and symptoms so you can be proactive in your health.

If a woman or girl suspects cancer, the physician will perform a biopsy to confirm or rule out cancer. If a biopsy is not possible, the doctor may suggest other tests that will help make a diagnosis. If cancer is diagnosed, more procedures such as an ultrasonography, computed tomography (CT), magnetic resonance imaging (MRI), x-rays may be done to determine the stage of the cancer. Staging is a way of describing where the cancer is located, if/where it has spread, and whether it is affecting the functions of other organs in the body. For all gynecologic cancers, stages range from I (the earliest) to IV (advanced). Within each stage, further distinction may be made. Identifying the stage of cancer helps the physician to decide what kind of treatment is best and can help predict a patient's prognosis, which is the chance of recovery.

Current treatments for most gynecological cancers, especially in advanced stages, usually include surgery followed by chemotherapy or a combination of chemo and radiation therapies. Chemotherapy may be given by injection, by mouth, or through a catheter inserted into the abdomen. How often chemotherapy is given depends on the type of cancer. Sometimes women have to remain at the hospital while they receive chemotherapy. When a gynecologic cancer is very advanced and a cure is not possible, radiation therapy or chemotherapy may still be recommended to reduce the size of the cancer or its metastases and to relieve pain and other symptoms. Relieving symptoms remains an important part of cancer care and treatment. This may also be called symptom management, palliative care, or supportive care.

Risk factors for gynecological cancers will vary from person to person. However, knowing your risk factors and talking about them with your physician will help you make more informed lifestyle and health care choices. The following factors affecting female reproductive system conditions include, but are not limited, to:

- age
- sexually transmitted infections (STIs), especially HPV.
- infection
- smoking
- immune system deficiency
- other female reproductive system health conditions
- genetics

- age at the time of first sexual intercourse
- social determinants such as poverty, lack of access to health care, or lack of insurance
- race and/or ethnicity

## Vulvovaginitis

At some point in a woman or girls reproductive years, she will develop an infection or excessive inflammation of the vagina or vulva tissues. This is a common condition called vulvovaginitis. Vulvovaginitis has a number of causes, including poor hygiene, bacteria, viruses, parasites, yeast, sexually transmitted diseases, exposure to allergens, chemical irritants, etc. Symptoms of vulvovaginitis can include vaginal itching, burning and inflammation, abnormal vaginal discharge, urinary discomfort or unpleasant vaginal odor. Vulvovaginitis is diagnosed by pelvic examination, which will involve collecting a sample of vaginal discharge to help determine which organism is causing the infection. Treatment of vulvovaginitis typically involves the use of antibiotic medications - oral or topical and behavioral changes that focuses on the underlying cause of the symptoms. The physician may also recommend a personal hygiene routine to help heal the infection and prevent it from recurring. Other suggestions may include wearing loose clothing and cotton underwear to allow the circulation of air and to reduce moisture. Removing underwear at bedtime may also help. Finally, avoiding bubble baths, perfumed soaps, and washing powders will also reduce the reoccurrence of vulvovaginitis.

### Vulvodynia

In the simplest of terms, vulvodynia means "pain of the vulva" without an identifiable cause. It is estimated to affect up to 16% of women and girls. Vulvodynia is chronic vulvar discomfort or pain, characterized by burning, stinging, irritation, or rawness of the female genitalia that last at least three (3) months.

There are two main subtypes of vulvodynia: 1) generalized vulvodynia and 2) localized vulvodynia also known as provoked vestibulodynia, formerly known as vulvar vestibulitis. Generalized vulvodynia is pain occurs spontaneously and is relatively constant, but there can be some periods of symptom relief. Localized vulvodynia/ vestibulodynia is characterized by pain limited to the vestibule, the area surrounding the opening of the vagina. Pain usually occurs during or after pressure is applied to the vestibule e.g. sexual intercourse, tampon insertion, a gynecologic examination, prolonged sitting, etc. In rare cases, the pain of vulvodynia may extend into the clitoris; this is referred to as clitorodynia.

The type of vulvodynia and severity of symptoms experienced are highly individualized. The most commonly reported symptom is burning, but women and girls descriptions of the pain vary. Vulvodynia, both localized and generalized, can have a huge impact on a woman's life. The pain can be so severe that it puts limitations on the ability to function and engage in daily activities such as work, tampon insertion, gynecological exams, sexual intercourse, or physical activities. Other complications of vulvodynia include shame, fear of having sex, anxiety, depression, sleep disturbances, body image issues, relationship problems, decreased quality of life, etc.

Vulvodynia is not caused by an active infection or a sexually transmitted disease. Researchers speculate that one or more of the following may cause, or contribute to, vulvodynia:

- irritation of, the nerves that transmit pain from the vulva
- increase in the number and sensitivity of pain-sensing nerve fibers in the vulva
- elevated levels of inflammatory substances in the vulva
- abnormal response of different types of vulvar cells to environmental factors such as infection or trauma
- genetics
- pelvic floor muscle weakness, spasm or instability

Vulvodynia is usually diagnosed after examinations of the vulvar site. During this exam, the physician will use the "cotton swab test" to differentiate between generalized and localized pain, delineate the areas of pain, and categorize their severity. During the examination, he or she will also conduct a thorough medical history including a complete blood work up and examination or vaginal fluids, to rule out infections or skin disorders. Once a physician has evaluated the symptoms, he or she can recommend treatments to help manage pain.

Treatment of vulvodynia requires a multidisciplinary approach since vulvodynia is not simply a gynecological condition. Effective treatment may involve visiting a gynecologist, sex therapist, pelvic floor therapist, neurologist, pain management specialist, etc. Because the exact causes of vulvodynia are unknown, treatments are directed towards alleviating symptoms and usually provides moderate pain relief. Effective treatment options may include a combination of lifestyle and behavioral changes, sex therapy, medications, pelvic floor exercises, vaginal dilation or surgery. No single treatment is appropriate for all women with vulvodynia and it may take time to find a treatment, or combination of treatments, that works for you.

Ovarian Cysts

Ovarian cysts are sac-like structures within or on the surface of the ovary that are filled with a fluid. Between eight and eighteen percent of women will develop ovarian cysts at some point during their lives. Ovarian cysts are common, especially with adolescent girls and woman who have menstrual cycles. Most ovarian cysts present little or no discomfort and are harmless, unless they increase in size or rupture. Most ovarian cysts are not cancerous; however, the risk does tend to rise as a woman gets older. Postmenopausal women with ovarian cysts are at higher risk for ovarian cancer.

Although there are various types of ovarian cysts, functional cysts are the most common type. Functional cysts are considered a result of the natural function of the menstrual cycle. There are two types of functional cysts: follicle and corpus luteum cysts.

**Follicle cyst:** During the menstrual cycle, an egg grows in a sac called a follicle. This sac is located inside the ovaries. In most cases, this follicle opens and releases an egg. However, if the follicle does not open to release the egg, the fluid inside the follicle forms a cyst on the ovary. Follicle cysts often have no symptoms and go away in one to three months.

**Corpus luteum cyst:** When a follicle sac releases its egg, the ruptured follicle sac begins to shrink and produce large quantities of estrogen and progesterone for conception. This follicle sac is now called the corpus luteum. If the sac does not shrink, additional fluid can build up inside the sac. This build up can become a cyst. Most corpus luteum cysts disappear within a few weeks.

Other types of ovarian cysts types of cysts are not related to the normal function of your menstrual cycle include:

**Dermoid cysts:** These cysts usually grow from cells that produce human eggs and may contain tissue, such as hair, skin, or teeth. They are rarely cancerous.

**Cystadenomas.** These non-cancerous cysts develop on the outer surface of the ovaries. They develop from ovarian tissue and may be filled with a watery liquid or a mucous material. These types of cysts are often attached to an ovary by a stalk rather than growing within the ovary itself.

**Endometriomas.** These cysts develop from endometriosis. The tissues that normally grow inside the uterus can develop outside the uterus and attach to the ovaries, resulting in a cyst.

Some women and girls develop a condition called **polycystic ovary syndrome,** or PCOS. This condition means the ovaries contain a large number of small cysts. The cysts develop due to a problem with ovulation, caused by a hormonal imbalance. PCOS can cause the ovaries to enlarge, and if left untreated, PCOS can lead to problems with menstruation, reduced fertility, hair growth, obesity, and acne.

To identify the type of cyst, the physician may order a pregnancy test. A positive pregnancy test may suggest that the cyst is a corpus luteum cyst. A pelvic ultrasound will help identify the location of the cyst and determine whether it is filled with fluid, mixed or solid. A laparoscopy will allow the physician to see the ovaries and remove the ovarian cyst, if needed. A blood test will check the level of protein called cancer antigen (CA 125) in the blood to determine whether the cyst could be cancerous. Women with ovarian cancer often have elevated levels of CA 125. Elevated CA 125 levels can also occur in noncancerous female reproductive conditions, such as endometriosis, uterine fibroids, and pelvic inflammatory disease.

Most ovarian cysts are small and do not cause symptoms. If a cyst does cause symptoms, the most common are pressure, bloating, swelling, or pain in the lower abdomen on the side of the cyst. This pain may be sharp or dull and may come and go. Less common symptoms include:

- pelvic pain
- dull ache in the lower back and thighs
- problems emptying the bladder or bowel completely
- pain during sexual intercourse
- unexplained weight gain
- pain during your period

- unusual vaginal bleeding
- breast tenderness
- needing to urinate more often
- pain during bowel movements or pressure on the bowels
- nausea or vomiting
- fullness or heaviness in the abdomen

If you have the following symptoms, please seek immediate medical care — these signs could mean your cyst has caused the ovary to twist or rupture:

- sudden, severe belly pain
- pain with fever and throwing up
- dizziness, weakness, feeling faint
- increased breathing

An ovarian cyst is typically found during a routine pelvic exam. Your doctor may notice swelling of one of the ovaries. If a cyst is suspected based upon symptoms or physical examination, the physician will utilize imaging techniques to confirm, determine the type of cyst and whether you need treatment. Most cysts are diagnosed by a pelvic or transvaginal ultrasound.

Most ovarian cysts are benign and naturally go away on their own without treatment. Because the majority of cysts disappear after a few weeks or months, a physician may not immediately recommend a treatment plan. Instead, he or she will watch and observe the cysts for any changes. If he or she observes any changes, they will move forward with more testing and treatment. To help determine the most effective treatment options, typically physicians will consider several factors such: size, location, whether or not the cyst is fluid filled or solid, whether or not it is producing any symptoms, and the woman/girls age. The treatment of an ovarian cyst may range from pain management of symptoms, to birth control pills, to surgical treatment.

Although there is no way to prevent the development of ovarian cysts, regular annual gynecologic examinations can help to detect any changes in ovaries. Keep in mind that symptoms of ovarian cancer can mimic symptoms of an ovarian cyst; therefore, it is extremely important to talk to your physician if you are experiencing any symptoms or changes that concern you.

## Yeast Infection

A vaginal yeast infection is a common infection that many women will experience at some point in their lifetime. It is a fungal infection that causes inflammation, irritation, discharge, and intense itchiness of the vagina and the vulva. Although a vaginal yeast infection is not considered a sexually transmitted infection, it can spread through mouth and genital contact.

The vagina naturally contains a balanced mix of yeast, including candida, and bacteria. The most common organism that causes yeast infections is known as Candida albicans. This type of yeast can be present in the vaginal canal without causing any symptoms at all. It is only when an overgrowth of this organism is present that the symptoms of a yeast infection may manifest. This happens when the balance of protective bacteria (lactobacillus bacteria) in the vagina is disturbed, due to either illness, hormonal changes, pregnancy, or taking certain medications, particularly antibiotics or immune-suppressing drugs. Conditions that affect the function of the immune system, including diabetes, can increase a woman's risk of getting a yeast infection.

Sometimes, other types of candida fungus are to blame. Common treatments usually cure a Candida albicans infection. Yeast infections caused by other types of candida fungus can be more difficult to treat, and need therapies that are more aggressive.

Yeast infection symptoms can range from mild to moderate and include:

- Itching and irritation in the vagina and the tissues at the vaginal opening
- A burning sensation, especially during intercourse or while urinating
- Redness and swelling of the vulva
- Vaginal pain and soreness
- Vaginal rash
- Watery vaginal discharge
- Thick, white, odor-free vaginal discharge with a cottage cheese appearance

Yeast infections are easy to treat, but it is important to see your physician if you think you have an infection. Yeast infection symptoms are similar to other vaginal infections and sexually transmitted infections (STIs).

To diagnose a yeast infection, your physician will perform a pelvic exam and examines your external and internal genitals for signs of infection. He or she may also send a sample of vaginal fluid for testing to determine the type of fungus causing the yeast infection. By identifying the type of fungus, the physician will be able to prescribe a more effective treatment, especially for reoccurring yeast infections.

Medications can effectively treat vaginal yeast infections. For mild to moderate symptoms and infrequent episodes of yeast infections, your doctor might recommend a short-course vaginal therapy that usually includes an anti-fungal regimen that lasts one, three or seven days or single dosage of oral medications. Treatment for a complicated yeast infection usually includes longer-course vaginal therapy of medications for seven to 14 days or multi dosage of oral medications. Treatment for recurrent yeast infections — four or more within a year — requires a longer treatment course and a maintenance plan. Maintenance therapy starts after a yeast infection is cleared with treatment. Therapies may include a regimen of oral tablets or vaginal suppositories once a week for six months. Additionally, if the sex partner is showing any signs of a genital yeast infection, the physician may recommend treatment for the partner.

**Q. Is it safe to use over-the-counter medicines for yeast infections?**
A. Always talk with your physician before treating yourself for a vaginal yeast infection. This is because you may be trying to treat an infection that is not a yeast infection, but a sexually transmitted infection (STIs) or another type of vaginal infection such as bacterial vaginosis (BV). STIs and

BV require different treatments than yeast infections and, if left untreated, can cause serious health problems. Additionally, using a yeast infection treatment when you do not actually have a yeast infection can cause your body to become resistant to the yeast infection medicine, which can make actual yeast infections harder to treat in the future.

**Q. IF I HAVE A YEAST INFECTION, DOES MY SEXUAL PARTNER NEED TO BE TREATED?**
A. Although yeast infections are not STIs, it is still possible to pass yeast infections to your partner during unprotected vaginal, oral, or anal sex. If your partner is a man, the risk of infection is low. However, research shows that about 15% of men get an itchy rash on the penis if they have unprotected sex with a woman who has a yeast infection. Men who have not been circumcised and men with diabetes are at increased risk. If your partner is a woman, she may be at risk. She should be tested and treated if she has any symptoms.

**Q. I HEARD THAT YOGURT PREVENTS OR TREATS YEAST INFECTIONS. IS THIS TRUE?**
A. Studies suggest that eating eight ounces of yogurt with "live cultures" daily can help prevent a yeast infection; however, more research still needs to be done to determine if yogurt with Lactobacillus or other probiotics can prevent or treat vaginal yeast infections.

*PEARLS OF WISDOM*
*Taking the following precautions can help to lower your risk of getting yeast infections:*

- *Do not douche. Douching removes some of the "good" bacteria in the vagina that protects it from infection*

- *Do not use scented feminine products.*

- *Change tampons, pads, and panty liners frequently.*

- *Do not wear tight underwear, pantyhose, pants, or jeans. These can increase body heat and moisture in your genital area and yeast thrives in moist environments.*

- *Wear underwear with a cotton crotch. Wearing cotton underwear does not hold in warmth and moisture.*

- *Change out of wet swimsuits and workout clothes as soon as possible.*

- *Always wipe from front to back.*

- *Reduce time in hot tubs and very hot baths.*

- *If you have diabetes, be sure your blood sugar is under control.*

## Pelvic Inflammatory Disease (PID)

Pelvic inflammatory disease, otherwise known as PID, is an infection that affects the organs female reproductive system, uterus, fallopian tubes, and ovaries. It is estimated to affect around 1 million women and girls every year in the United States.

PID is usually caused by an untreated a bacteria sexually transmitted infection such as chlamydia or gonorrhea that spreads from the vagina and cervix.

Symptoms of PID range from none to severe. Symptoms of PID include:

- pain in your lower belly
- heavy discharge vaginal discharge with an unpleasant odor
- unexplained bleeding between periods
- irregular periods
- pain during intercourse

- fever and/or chills
- pain when urinating
- infertility
- ectopic pregnancy

Symptoms of PID can mimic other medical conditions and can be life threatening, therefore it is extremely important to consult a physician right away if you are experiencing any symptoms.

PID is more common in adolescent girls ages 15- 24. Additionally, young women with multiple sex partners are at greatest risk for pelvic inflammatory disease. Douching and a history of PID increase the chances of being infected with PID. Douching can push bacteria into the reproductive organs and can hide the signs of PID.

If PID is suspected, a physician will do a pelvic exam, an analysis of vaginal discharge and cervical cultures, or urinary analysis. To confirm the diagnosis or to determine how widespread the infection is other test such as imaging methods, such as ultrasonography - pelvic or vaginal, computed tomography (CT), and magnetic imaging (MRI), can aid in diagnosis. In the case of severe symptoms, a physician may also an endometrial biopsy and laparoscopy.

Antibiotics are used to treat PID. It is important to take all the antibiotics according to how it is prescribe, even if your symptoms go away. This helps to make sure the infection is fully cured. Failure to do so may make the condition worse and require further treatment. If there is no improvement within two to three days, the patient is typically advised to seek further medical attention.

Hospitalization sometimes becomes necessary if there are other complications of treatment.

Although PID can be treated, the treatment will not undo any damage that has already happened to your reproductive system. The longer you wait to be treated, the more likely it is that you will have complications from PID. Additionally, if a woman or girl is being treated for PID, the physician may recommend that her sex partner (s) be treated as well.

PID can be prevented by practicing safer sex, i.e. condoms and dental dams, reducing the number of sex partners, practicing abstinence, and being in a mutually monogamous relationship. Ways to reduce risk will be discussed in more detail later in the book.

# CHAPTER 6:

# SEXUALLY TRANSMITTED INFECTIONS OF THE FEMALE REPRODUCTIVE SYSTEM

Having a sexually transmitted infection (STI) can definitely have an impact on sexual pleasure. An STI can cause significant pain to your internal and external sex organs. This pain may intensify during intercourse. STI's can also be tricky. Some STIs, particularly gonorrhea and chlamydia, may not show any symptoms until it is too late or until it causes scarring and major damage to an organ. Additionally, some STIs will cause vaginal itching and dryness, which may also make sex painful.

According to United Sates Department of Health and Human Services, about 19 million new sexually transmitted infections are thought to occur each year. These infections affect women of all backgrounds and economic levels.

There more than 30 different bacteria, viruses, and parasites which can cause an STI. Bacterial STIs include chlamydia, gonorrhea, syphilis, and bacterial vaginosis. Viral STIs include genital herpes, hepatitis B, HPV and HIV. Parasitic STIs include Trichomoniasis.

## CHLAMYDIA

Chlamydia is one of the most common STIs. It affects approximately 4 million women annually. Because symptoms of chlamydia are not always apparent, it is not easy to tell if a woman is infected with chlamydia – when they do occur, they are usually noticeable within one to three weeks of contact and can include the following:

- abnormal vaginal discharge that may have an odor
- bleeding between periods
- painful periods
- abdominal pain with fever pain when having sex
- itching or burning in or around the vagina
- pain when urinating

Chlamydia can be detected on material collected by swabbing the cervix during a traditional examination using a speculum. Treatment of chlamydia involves antibiotics. A convenient single-dose therapy for chlamydia is oral azithromycin. Alternative treatments are often used, however, because of the high cost of this medication. The most common alternative treatment is doxycycline. If left untreated, chlamydia infection can cause pelvic inflammatory disease, which can lead to damage of the fallopian tubes (the tubes connecting the ovaries to the uterus) or even cause infertility (the inability to have children). Untreated chlamydia infection could also increase the risk of ectopic pregnancy.

Chlamydia can be cured with the right treatment. Treatment of chlamydia involves antibiotics. A convenient, single-dose therapy for chlamydia is oral azithromycin. Alternative treatments are often used, however, because of the high cost of this medication. The most common alternative treatment is doxycycline. If left untreated, chlamydia infection can cause pelvic inflammatory disease, which can lead to damage of the fallopian tubes (the tubes connecting the ovaries to the uterus), or even cause infertility (the inability to have children). Untreated chlamydia infection could also increase the risk of ectopic pregnancy.

## GONORRHEA

Gonorrhea, which is caused by a bacterium, is one of the oldest known sexually transmitted diseases. It is estimated that over one million women are currently infected with gonorrhea. Among women who are infected, a significant percentage also will be infected with chlamydia. Gonorrhea can only survive on moist surfaces within the body and is found most commonly in the vagina, and, more commonly, the cervix. It can also live in the urethra, back of the throat and in the rectum. A majority of infected women have no symptoms, especially in the early stages of the infection. When they do occur, they are usually noticeable within one to three weeks of contact and can include the following:

- burning or frequent urination
- yellowish vaginal discharge
- redness and swelling of the genitals
- burning or itching of the vaginal area

Like Chlamydia, gonorrhea can lead to a severe pelvic infection with inflammation of the Fallopian tubes and ovaries, also known as pelvic inflammatory disease (PID)

Testing for gonorrhea is done by swabbing the infected site (rectum, throat, or cervix) and identifying the bacteria in the laboratory either through culturing of the material from the swab (growing the bacteria) or identification of the genetic material from the bacteria. In the past, the treatment of uncomplicated gonorrhea was fairly simple. A single injection of penicillin cured almost every infected person. Unfortunately, there are new strains of gonorrhea that have become resistant to various antibiotics, including penicillin, and are therefore more difficult to treat. Fortunately, gonorrhea can still be treated by other injectable or oral medications. The sexual partners of women who have had either gonorrhea or chlamydia must receive treatment for both infections since their partners may be infected as well. Treating the partners also prevents reinfection of the woman. Women suffering from PID may require more aggressive treatment that is effective against the bacteria that cause gonorrhea as well as against other organisms. These women often require intravenous (IV) administration of antibiotics.

## SYPHILIS

Syphilis is an STD that has been around for centuries. It is caused by a bacterial organism called a spirochete. The spirochete is a wormlike, spiral-shaped organism that wiggles vigorously when viewed under a microscope. It infects the person by burrowing into the moist, mucous-covered lining of the mouth or genitals. Symptoms in adults are divided into stages. These stages are primary, secondary, latent, and late syphilis.

Syphilis has been called 'the great imitator' because it has so many possible symptoms, many of which look like symptoms from other diseases.

### Primary Stage

During the first (primary) stage of syphilis, you may notice a single sore, but there may be multiple sores. The sore is the location where syphilis entered your body. The sore is usually firm, round, and painless. Because the sore is painless, it can easily go unnoticed. The sore lasts 3 to 6 weeks. In most women, an early infection resolves on its own, even without treatment. Even though the sore goes away, you must still receive treatment so your infection does not move to the secondary stage.

### Secondary Stage

During the secondary stage, you may have skin rashes and/or sores in your mouth, vagina, or anus. This stage usually starts with a rash on one or more areas of your body. The rash usually will not itch and it is sometimes so faint that you won't notice it. Other symptoms you may have can include fever, swollen lymph glands, sore throat, patchy hair loss, headaches, weight loss, muscle aches, and fatigue (feeling very tired). The symptoms from this stage will go away whether or not you receive treatment. Without the right treatment, your infection will move to the latent and possibly late stages of syphilis.

### Latent and Late Stages

The latent stage of syphilis begins when all of the symptoms you had earlier disappear. If you do not receive treatment, you can continue to have syphilis in your body for years without any signs or symptoms. Most people with untreated syphilis do not develop late stage syphilis. However, when late stage syphilis does occur, it is very serious and would appear 10–30 years after your infection began. Symptoms of the late stage of syphilis include difficulty coordinating your muscle movements, paralysis (unable to move parts of your body), numbness, blindness, and dementia (mental disorder). In the late stages of syphilis, the disease damages your internal organs and can result in death.

Syphilis can be diagnosed by scraping the base of the ulcer and looking under a special type of microscope (dark field microscope) for the spirochetes. Special blood tests can also be used to diagnose syphilis. The blood test detect the body's response to the infection, but not to the actual Treponema organism that causes the infection. Syphilis can be cured with the right antibiotics from your health care provider. However, treatment will not undo any damage that the infection has already done.

Depending on the stage of disease, the treatment options for syphilis vary. Penicillin injections have been very effective in treating both early and late stage syphilis. Alternative treatments for syphilis may include oral doxycycline or tetracycline.

## BACTERIAL VAGINOSIS

Bacterial vaginosis (BV) is not typically considered a sexually transmitted infection, because some experts feel it can occur in women who are not sexually active. Bacterial vaginosis is the overgrowth or imbalance of certain bacteria within the vagina, leading in some cases to symptoms including a vaginal discharge that may be foul smelling. Although bacterial vaginosis is found in women of all ages, it is most common vaginal infection in the US in women of childbearing age. BV is caused by an imbalance of the naturally occurring bacteria in the vagina. Like many other STI, Most women with bacterial vaginosis do not have symptoms from the condition. When symptoms are present, they include:

- abnormal vaginal discharge
- fishy odor
- vaginal itching and burning
- burning during urination

The best way to diagnose bacterial vaginosis is examination of the vaginal discharge under a microscope by finding a higher than normal vaginal pH and large numbers of bacteria. A pelvic exam, including diagnostic tests for other causes of symptoms, such as gonorrhea and chlamydia, may also be performed at the time of diagnosis. Some of cases of bacterial vaginosis will clear up without any treatment. Nevertheless, treatment with antibiotics is recommended. Metronidazole may be given orally in pill form or applied as a vaginal gel.

## GENITAL HERPES

Genital herpes, also commonly called "herpes," is a viral infection by the herpes simplex virus (HSV) that is transmitted through intimate contact with the mucous-covered linings of the mouth or the vagina or the genital skin. In the United States, about one out of every six people aged 14 to 49 years have genital herpes. The virus enters the linings or skin through microscopic tears. Once inside, the virus travels to the nerve roots near the spinal cord and settles there permanently. When an infected person has a herpes outbreak, the virus travels down the nerve fibers to the site of the original infection. When it reaches the skin, the typical redness and blisters occur. After the initial outbreak, subsequent outbreaks tend to be sporadic. They may occur weekly or even years apart.

Two types of herpes viruses are associated with genital lesions: herpes simplex virus-1 (HSV-1) and herpes simplex virus-2 (HSV-2). HSV-1 more often causes blisters of the mouth area while HSV-2 more often causes genital sores or lesions in the area around the anus. The outbreak of herpes is closely related to the functioning of the immune system. Women who have suppressed immune systems, because of stress, infection, or medications, have more frequent and longer-lasting outbreaks.

Genital herpes is spread only by direct person-to-person contact. It is believed that a majority of sexually active adults carry the herpes virus. Part of the reason for the continued high infection rate is that most women infected with the herpes virus do not know that they are infected because they have few or no symptoms.

Once exposed to the virus, an incubation period generally lasts three to seven days before a lesion develops. During this time, there are no symptoms and the virus cannot be transmitted to others. An outbreak usually begins within two weeks of initial infection and manifests as an itching or tingling sensation followed by redness of the skin. Finally, a blister forms. The blisters and subsequent ulcers that form when the blisters break, are usually very painful to touch and may last from seven days to two weeks. The infection is definitely contagious from the time of itching to the time of complete healing of the ulcer, usually within two to four weeks. However, as noted above, infected individuals can also transmit the virus to their sex partners in the absence of a recognized outbreak.

Only a health care provider can diagnose herpes by performing a physical exam and tests. A blood test can tell if you are infected with oral or genital herpes, even if you don't have symptoms. Genital herpes is suspected when multiple painful blisters occur in a sexually exposed area. During the initial outbreak, fluid from the blisters may be sent to the laboratory to culture the virus. There are also blood tests that can detect antibodies to the herpes viruses

Although there is no known cure for herpes, there are treatments for the outbreaks. Treatments can be are oral medications, such as acyclovir (Zovirax) or topical which are applied directly on the lesions.

## HEPATITIS B

Hepatitis B virus (HBV) is a virus that causes inflammation of the liver. Most people do not think of hepatitis as a sexually transmitted infection; however, one of the more common modes of the spread of viral hepatitis B is through intimate sexual contact. Hepatitis B is spread through semen, vaginal fluids, blood, and urine. About 46,000 American women, men, and children become infected with HBV each year. Most of these infections occur among people who are age 20 to 49.

Because hepatitis B often has no symptoms, most people are not aware that they have the infection. One out of two adults who have it never have hepatitis B symptoms. When hepatitis B symptoms do occur, they usually appear between six weeks and six months after infection. When hepatitis B symptoms do develop, the ones most likely to happen first include:

- extreme tiredness
- tenderness and pain in the lower abdomen
- loss of appetite
- nausea, vomiting
- pain in the joints
- headache
- fever
- hives
- severe abdominal pain
- dark urine
- pale-colored bowel movements
- jaundice

Hepatitis B is usually diagnosed by detecting antibodies against the virus and by blood tests that identify the virus in the blood. There is no cure for HBV. HBV usually gets better on its own after a few months. If it does not get better, it is called chronic HBV, which lasts a lifetime.

Chronic HBV can lead to scarring of the liver, liver failure, or liver cancer.

Although there is no cure for HBV, it can be treated. Acute hepatitis, unless severe, needs no treatment. Some patients with chronic hepatitis may be treated with antiviral drugs. These medicines can decrease or remove hepatitis B from the blood. They also help to reduce the risk of cirrhosis and liver cancer. If you develop liver failure, a liver transplant is the only cure in some cases of liver failure.

A highly effective vaccine that prevents hepatitis B is currently available. It is recommended that all babies be vaccinated against HBV beginning at birth, and all children under the age of 18 who have not been vaccinated should also receive the vaccination. Among adults, anyone who wishes to do so may receive the vaccine, and it is recommended especially for anyone whose behavior or lifestyle may pose a risk of HBV infection.

## Human papillomavirus (HPV)

HPV infection is now considered the most common sexually transmitted infection in the US, and it is believed that at a majority of the reproductive-age population has been infected with sexually transmitted HPV at some point in life. There are more than 40 different types of HPV — types that are transmitted through direct sexual contact, and types that are passed from the skin and mucous membranes of infected people to the skin and mucous membranes of their partners.

Some sexually transmitted HPV types may cause genital warts. Persistent infection with "high-risk" HPV types — different from the ones that cause skin warts — may progress to precancerous lesions and invasive cancer. High-risk HPV infection is a cause of nearly all cases of cervical cancer. However, most infections do not cause disease. Most high-risk HPV infections occur without any symptoms, go away within one to two years, and do not cause cancer. Some HPV infections, however, can persist for many years. Persistent infections with high-risk HPV types can lead to cell changes that, if untreated, may progress to cancer.

Genital warts usually appear as small, fleshy, raised bumps, but they can sometimes be extensive and have a cauliflower-like appearance. In many cases, genital warts do not cause any symptoms, but they are sometimes associated with itching, burning, or tenderness.

HPV can usually be diagnosed by the presence of warts on the genital area. HPV can sometimes be suspected by changes that appear on a Pap smear, although Pap smears were not really designed to detect HPV.

In the case of an abnormal Pap smear, the health care professional will often do advanced testing on the cells to determine if to see if they contain viral DNA or RNA. HPV can also be detected if a biopsy is sent to the laboratory for analysis. An appearance of a genital lesion may prompt the physician to treat without further testing.

There is currently no medical treatment for HPV. However, the health problems caused by HPV (genital warts, precancerous changes at the cervix, and cancers resulting from HPV infections) can be treated. If one partner has genital warts, avoid having sex until the warts are gone or removed.

Currently, there are three vaccines approved to help prevent HPV infection. These vaccines provide strong protection against new HPV infections. HPV vaccinations given before sexual activity can reduce the risk of infection by the HPV types targeted by the vaccine. However, they are not effective at treating established HPV infections or disease caused by HPV. In addition, these vaccines are still too new to determine the long-term implications on the body. If you are interested in learning more about the vaccine, talk with your health care professional to determine if the vaccine is right for you.

## TRICHOMONIASIS

Trichomoniasis, sometimes referred to as "trich," is a common STD that affects two to three million Americans yearly. It is caused by a single-celled protozoan parasite called Trichomonas vaginalis. Trichomoniasis is primarily an infection of the urogenital tract; the urethra is the most common site of infection in man, and the vagina is the most common site of infection in women. Trichomoniasis, like many other STIs, often occurs without any symptoms. When and if symptoms appear, usually within four to twenty days of exposure, they include:

- heavy, yellow-green or gray vaginal discharge
- discomfort during intercourse
- vaginal odor
- painful urination
- abdominal pain
- vaginal itching and irritation

- painful sex

Trichomoniasis is usually diagnosed by a physical examination and lab test. Lab tests are performed on a sample of vaginal fluid or urethral fluid to look for the disease-causing parasite.

The oral antibiotic metronidazole is used to treat women with Trichomoniasis. It usually is administered orally in a single dose. Your partner should also be treated at the same time to prevent reinfection and further spread of the disease. In addition, persons being treated for Trichomoniasis should avoid sex until they and their sex partners complete treatment and have no symptoms. It is important to take all of your antibiotics, even if you feel better.

Having an STI can definitely have an impact on reproductive health and even sexual pleasure. An STI can cause significant pain to your internal and external reproductive organs. This pain may intensify during intercourse. STIs can also be tricky. Some STIs, particularly gonorrhea and chlamydia, may not show any symptoms until it is too late or until it causes scarring and major damage to an organ. Additionally, some STIs will cause vaginal itching and dryness that may also make the genital are pretty painful. If you suspect that you have an STI, it is important to be evaluated as soon as possible to relieve the pain and/or reduce the chances of infertility. I will discuss how to protect yourself and reduce the risk of getting an STI in more detail in the following chapter.

## Human Immunodeficiency Virus

HIV stands for human immunodeficiency virus.

**H** – Human – This particular virus can only infect human beings.

**I** – Immunodeficiency – HIV weakens your immune system by destroying important cells that fight disease and infection. A "deficient" immune system can't protect you.

**V** – Virus – A virus can only reproduce itself by taking over a cell in the body of its host.

Currently, there is no cure for HIV/AIDS, but there are medications that can dramatically slow disease progression. **Once you have HIV, you will have it for life.**

What is AIDS?

AIDS" stands for Acquired Immunodeficiency Syndrome. To understand what that means, let's break it down:

**A** – Acquired – AIDS is not something you inherit from your parents. You acquire AIDS after birth.

**I** – Immuno – Your body's immune system includes all the organs and cells that work to fight off infection or disease.

**D** – Deficiency – You get AIDS when your immune system is "deficient," or isn't working the way it should.

**S** – Syndrome – A syndrome is a collection of symptoms and signs of disease. AIDS is a syndrome, rather than a single disease, because it is a complex illness with a wide range of complications and symptoms.

Once a person receives a diagnosis of AIDS, it means that he or she has met a predetermined set of criteria as defined by a doctor: 1) You are considered to have progressed to AIDS if you have one or more specific opportunistic infections, or 2) the CD4 cells have fallen below 200. Only a doctor can diagnose someone as having AIDS.

## What Happens when HIV Enters the Body?

When HIV enters the body, it attacks a key part of your immune system – your T-cells or CD4 cells. HIV invades the cells and uses them to make more copies of itself, and then destroys them. Normally, our body has the ability to fight infections and disease, but a person with a compromised immune system cannot fight off HIV.

During the initial onset, or primary/acute infection of HIV, usually two to eight weeks, the majority of people develop flu-like symptoms after the virus enters the body. This illness, known as primary or acute HIV infection, may last for a few weeks. Possible signs and symptoms include:

- fever
- headache
- muscle aches
- rash
- chills
- sore throat
- mouth or genital ulcers
- swollen lymph glands, mainly on the neck
- joint pain

- night sweats
- diarrhea

Although the symptoms of primary HIV infection may be mild enough to go unnoticed, and or not be detected on an HIV test, the amount of virus in the bloodstream (viral load) is particularly high at this time and HIV can be spread if an individual is engaging in risky behaviors.

It is important to know that even though the level of the virus may be low or have an undetectable viral load, this does not mean that a person no longer has HIV or that they cannot transmit HIV.

Viral load refers to the amount of HIV in an infected person's blood. An undetectable viral load is when the amount of HIV in a person's blood is so low that it can't be measured. However, a person with HIV can still potentially transmit HIV to a partner even if they have an undetectable viral load, because:

- HIV may still be found in a person's genital fluids (e.g., semen, vaginal fluids). The viral load test only measures virus in a person's blood.
- A person's viral load may go up between tests. When this happens, they may be more likely to transmit HIV to partners.
- Sexually transmitted diseases (STDs) increase viral load in a person's genital fluids.

Another particular danger during the initial onset of acute infection period is that because the signs and symptoms mimic many other conditions, most people assume they have the flu, treat the signs and symptoms with over-the-counter meds, and/or ignore the symptoms. The danger in this is that they do not test for HIV unless they know for sure that they have put themselves at risk for HIV.

After the initial onset of acute infection period, the immune system loses the battle with HIV and symptoms go away. HIV infection goes into its second stage, which can be a long period without symptoms, called the asymptomatic (or latent) period. This is when people may not know they are infected and can pass HIV on to others. This period can last 10 or more years. During this period without symptoms, HIV is slowly killing the CD4 T-cells and destroying the immune system.

Over time, HIV destroys so many of your T-cells that the immune system begins to break down. When that happens, HIV infection can lead to the third and final stage of HIV, an AIDS diagnosis. However, not everyone who has HIV will progress to AIDS. With proper treatment and adherence to medical protocols, an individual infected with HIV can keep the level of HIV in their body low.

**What Are the Fluids That Transmit HIV?**
HIV is transmitted by coming in contact with certain body fluids of a person that is infected with HIV. These body fluids are:

- Blood
- Semen (cum)
- Pre-seminal fluid (pre-cum)
- Vaginal fluids

- Breast milk

These body fluids must come into contact with a mucous membrane or damaged tissue or be directly injected into your bloodstream (by a needle or syringe) for transmission to possibly occur. Mucous membranes are the soft, moist areas just inside the openings to your body such as the inside the rectum, the vagina or the opening of the penis, and the mouth.

HIV is most commonly diagnosed by testing your blood or saliva for antibodies and/or the virus. Most people who are tested for HIV will show an accurate result after about two to eight weeks from infection. In rare cases, it may take up to six months for enough HIV antibodies to build up in the blood to be detected on an HIV antibody test. **Currently, there is no cure for HIV, only treatment.** Early HIV antiretroviral treatment is crucial—it improves quality of life, extends life expectancy and reduces the risk of transmission.

# CHAPTER 7:

# OTHER CONCERNS OF THE FEMALE REPRODUCTIVE SYSTEM

In addition to some of the common reproductive health conditions and sexually transmitted infections, other things can cause significant discomfort and/or irritate the vulva and vagina.

## DIET

The type of diet a woman or girl has can influence that pH of the vagina—including smell and taste. A diet high in sugars, starches, and processed foods increase chances that the environment of the vagina will be compromised. The reason it is important to reduce your intake of sugars, starches and processed foods is because they are a primary source of food for fungus and parasites that reside in your vagina. A balanced, nutritious diet of fruits, nuts, vegetables and plenty of water are key to vaginal and reproductive health. A healthy diet can also help improve the smell and taste of your vagina.

## ALLERGIES

### Semen

A sperm allergy is a rare allergic reaction to the proteins found in a man's semen, which mostly affects women. For some women, the symptoms may be localized—affecting the only the area that has come in contact with the semen i.e., vagina, mouth, anus, or skin. For others, the symptoms can affect their entire body. Some common symptoms of sperm allergy are redness, swelling, pain, itching, and a burning sensation in the vaginal area. In rare cases, a woman may have hives, swelling, trouble breathing, or anaphylaxis, a life-threatening allergic reaction. Symptoms usually start about 10-30 minutes after contact with semen. Symptoms can last for a few hours or a few days. The onset can vary. A woman could have been just fine with a partner's semen for a couple of years, and then suddenly start having an allergic reaction to it for no good reason. Additionally, a sperm allergy may also occur with one partner but not another. A sperm allergy is often misdiagnosed as vaginitis (inflammation of the vagina), a yeast infection, or a sexually transmitted infection (STI). The major determining for diagnosis is condom use. The allergic reaction should only happen during unprotected sex. If a sperm allergy is suspected, the physician may refer to an allergist to a skin test with the partner's semen to confirm the allergy. In the case of pregnancy, a woman with a sperm allergy can still get pregnant through artificial insemination or in vitro fertilization, after sperm is washed.

### Latex

In the United States, approximately one to three percent of people are allergic to latex. An allergy to latex can cause vaginal irritation, burning, itching, redness, and blistering. In rare cases, an allergic reaction to latex may cause anaphylactic shock, which requires immediate medical attention. Symptoms of anaphylactic shock include shortness of breath, feeling faint, nausea, hives, and fainting. A reaction to latex usually occurs within a day and can last up to four days. A latex allergy is usually diagnosed by ruling out other sources of irritation such as an STI. The physician may also refer you to an allergist who can do a blood test to determine your latex sensitivity. Women or girls who are allergic to latex can use a condom made of polyisoprene (rubber) or polyurethane for sexual intercourse will help with latex allergy.

## SHAVING, TRIMMING AND WAXING

Shaving, trimming and waxing are popular practices especially among younger women, however it does not come without a risk. Women and/or girls who shave, trim, or wax their mons pubis and vulva may get folliculitis. Folliculitis appears as small, red, and sometimes painful bumps caused by bacteria that infect a hair follicle. The friction from clothing and sexual intercourse can cause further irritation to the genitals, creating a portal of entry for bacteria and other infections to enter the body. Folliculitis often goes away by itself. Attention to hygiene, wearing loose clothing, and warm compresses applied to the area can help speed up the healing process. If the bumps do not go away or they get bigger, see your physician for additional treatment.

## UNDERWEAR

I know we all want to experience Victoria's Secret; however, wearing the wrong type of underwear can irritate the vulva and increase your chance for getting an infection. Breathable, natural fabrics such as cotton are the best choice. If an all-cotton panty is not your thing, then at least wear a panty with a cotton crotch. Cotton allows the genitals to get proper ventilation, which helps to reduce moisture. Remember, bacteria likes to thrive in moist environments. If you like to wear thongs, please keep in mind that while thongs may be sexy, they create a direct pathway for moisture and bacteria in the anus to travel to the vulva and vagina, which increase the risk of infection.

## STRESS

Stress can be overwhelming and take a toll on us, not just mentally, emotionally, socially or spiritually, but physically as well. When we stress out, it affects the immunes system's ability to fight off infections. This reduces the body's natural pH, making us more susceptible to infections. Our body continuously strives to maintain a balanced pH within its fluids. Changes in vaginal pH because of stress can have harsh consequences, making the vagina far more vulnerable to problems such as odor, irritation, or even sexually transmitted infections.

## JEANS

Skinny jeans are trendy and cute but before you consider replacing all of your old jeans with skinny jeans, keep in mind that wearing jeans that are too tight can increase the risk for infections. Tight clothing can cause friction against sensitive genital tissues creating microscopic tears in the tissues. This opens up a portal of entry for bacteria to enter the body. In addition, tight jeans can trap moisture in the genital area creating the perfect breeding ground of a yeast infection.

## HYGIENE PRODUCTS

Many women have concerns about how their vagina smells. Contrary to popular belief, the vulva nor the vagina should smell like roses or springtime. In the United States alone, women and girls spend well over two billion per year on feminine hygiene products, including tampons, pads, feminine washes, sprays, powders, and personal wipes. While nearly all women and girls use tampons and sanitary pads, black and Latina women and girls use douches, wipes, powders, and deodorizers more often than women of other races. This puts them at greater risk of potential chemical exposures. The skin of the vulva is very delicate. As a mucous membrane, the vagina, vulva, including the clitoris, clitoral hood, labia minora, and urethra is capable of secreting and absorbing fluids at a higher rate than skin.

Many products contain chemicals like pesticides, glycerin, color additives, endocrine-disrupting chemicals (EDCs), carcinogens, or allergens that can cause irritation to the vagina and vulva. Some of these products include contraceptive forms or jellies, latex condoms, vaginal sprays and deodorants, scented tampons, perfumed body soaps and douches. This includes other products that come into contact with the genitals, such as tissue, laundry detergents, etc. These products can cause the vaginal lining to dry out making the vagina more prone to rips and tearing during intercourse. In addition, the products can cause inflammation, intense itching and burning to the vulva - **vulvovaginitis.** Only warm water and a mild soap (if absolutely necessary) should be used to wash the vulva, not the vagina. If there is a foul odor coming from the vagina, it does not mean that you need to use a product to try to get rid of the odor. Using a product will only mask the odor and/or make it much more apparent. A foul odor is an indication of an infection and you need to contact your physician immediately to determine the cause.

## INJECTIONS, IMPLANTS AND SUCH: ALTERING THE FEMALE GENITALIA

In recent years, we have seen a lot of celebrities (and even everyday women) undergoing procedures to alter their genitalia — ranging from bedazzling the mons pubis to vaginoplasty. Many of these women and girls are choosing to have such procedures because of the shame that society has placed on the genitalia of women and girls.

According to the American College of Obstetricians and Gynecologist (ACOG), the most common female genital surgeries are laser resurfacing of the labia to remove wrinkles, labiaplasty (reducing the size of the labia), vaginal tightening, vaginal rejuvenation, designer vaginoplasty, re-virgination, and G-spot amplification.

The safety of these procedures has not been documented. Women and girls seeking these surgeries need to be informed about the lack of data supporting these procedures and the potential associated risks such as infection, altered sensation, dyspareunia (difficult or painful sexual intercourse), adhesions, and scarring.

The heavy advertising in the media and the endorsements from celebrities for these procedures, in combination with a lack of public education, fosters body shame and insecurities on the genitalia of women and girls despite the fact that there are individual variations in the size, color, etc. of genitalia.

## LACK OF LUBRICATION AND VAGINAL DRYNESS

Normally, the lining of the vagina stay lubricated with a thin layer of clear fluid, however there are many things that can cause the lining to become dry. As the vagina's ability to make its own mucus declines, it can become irritated, itchy, and painful. Additionally, insufficient lubrication or vaginal dryness can cause mild to significant pain and interfere with sexual pleasure. Vaginal dryness is nothing to be embarrassed about. It affects many women, especially as they age.

Several things can affect a woman's ability to lubricate, resulting in vaginal dryness. Reduced estrogen levels are the main cause of vaginal dryness. Estrogen helps keep vaginal tissue healthy by maintaining normal vaginal lubrication, tissue elasticity, and acidity. These factors create a natural defense against vaginal and infections. However, when your estrogen levels decrease, so does this natural defense, leading to a thinner, less elastic and more fragile vaginal lining, and an increased risk of infections.

Additional causes of vaginal dryness include: pregnancy, lactation, menopause, aging, immune disorders, chemotherapy, sexually transmitted infections, smoking cigarette, perfumed soaps, bubble bath, flavored lubricants, douching will reduce lubrication and may cause the vagina to feel dry and irritated. In addition, certain medications will cause dryness, especially those with ingredients that will reduce moisture of the mucosal or "wet" tissues of the vagina. Such medicines include many common drugs for allergies, cardiovascular, psychiatric, and other medical conditions. Oral contraceptives may also decrease vaginal lubrication. Irritation from contraceptive creams and foams can also cause dryness, as can fear and anxiety about sexual intimacy

Vaginal dryness may also result from insufficient foreplay and arousal. In many cases, women need lots of sexual stimulation for arousal. The more aroused she is, the more likely her lubrication will increase, reducing dryness and friction as well as helping to make sexual intercourse more pleasure.

Vaginal dryness may be accompanied by signs and symptoms such as:

- Itching or stinging around the vaginal opening
- Burning
- Soreness
- Pain with intercourse
- Light bleeding with intercourse
- Urinary frequency or urgency
- Recurrent urinary tract infections
- Involuntary contractions of the pelvic floor muscles

If a woman is experiencing vaginal dryness, she should listen to her body. Vaginal dryness may be an indication that something is going on with her body and she needs to consult with her physician to determine the underlying cause of the dryness. In addition, boosting water intake by drinking at least ten 8-oz. glasses of water a day may help to relieve vaginal dryness. Following a hormone-balancing diet will provide the body the right nutritional support to make and balance your hormones.

If vaginal dryness is a problem during sexual intercourse, using a lubricant can help reduce the irritation. Vaginal lubricants can support and/or naturally restore your own vaginal moisture. Whether a woman has an issue or not with lubrication, it is always a good idea to keep lubrication nearby. The more the vagina is lubricated, the less likely the lining of the vaginal will have excessive ripping and tearing from intercourse. The more rips and tears in the vaginal helps to create a portal of entry for bacteria and other infections.

**Lubricants**. Water-based or silicone-based lubricants can help keep your vagina lubricated. Choose products that do not contain glycerin, which has been linked to yeast infections.

Moisturizers imitate normal vaginal moisture and relieve dryness for up to three days with a single application. Use these as ongoing protection from the irritation of vaginal dryness. Before using complementary or alternative treatments, such as vitamin therapies or products containing estrogen, talk to your physician first.

Natural and Organic Lubricants such as cosmetic grade oils such as almond, coconut or olive oils act as lubricants and can be helpful in rejuvenating irritated, dry tissues.

Keep in mind that while the use of a lubricant can make sexual intercourse less painful, it does not address the underlying cause of the vaginal dryness itself.

### Q. DURING INTERCOURSE, I GET REALLY DRY.

*Halfway through the session, it becomes very uncomfortable, and sometimes I have to ask my husband to stop. It really frustrates me because I do not understand what's going on. Dr. TaMara, can you please help me with this issue? I mean, I really love my husband, and he turns me on, but I do not want him to think he does not because I cannot stay wet.*

A. A woman's vagina naturally lubricates itself; however, when there is insufficient lubrication it can cause pain and interfere with sexual pleasure. When sex hurts, it can definitely damper the mood, the relationship and cause feelings of inadequacy. Please keep in mind that there is a difference between pain and discomfort. Discomfort is a feeling that may not be pleasurable but it is bearable. Pain is a feeling that is unbearable. Pain is an indication that something is wrong with your body and whatever it is that you are doing, you need to stop immediately before you do further damage. If you are experiencing any pain during sex, consider contacting your physician and/or your local sex therapist to get to the root of the problem. Finally, do not be embarrassed to whip out that lubricant! In addition to using a lubricant, perhaps try telling your partner how much you enjoy foreplay and that it really turns you on. Foreplay is helpful because it gets the blood flowing to the genitals. This helps to increase natural lubrication in the vagina. Remember there is a difference between arousal and desire. Arousal is a physiological response and desire is a psychological response. Just because your body may not be responding in the physical manner that you would like, you still desire him sexually. Consider explaining this to your husband as well.

Vaginal dryness is nothing to be embarrassed about. It affects many women, especially as they age. If vaginal dryness begins to affects your lifestyle, sex life and/or relationship with your partner; consider making an appointment with your physician. You do not have to live with uncomfortable vaginal dryness.

**Q. HOW COULD A REPRODUCTIVE SYSTEM HEALTH CONDITION IMPACT MY SEX LIFE?**
A. Sexual feelings and attitudes vary greatly among women, even when they do not have a reproductive health condition. Some women have little or no change in their sexual desire and energy level when they have a reproductive health

condition. Others find that they have less interest in sex because of their particular condition.

If your sexual desire and energy levels change after your diagnosis, keep in mind that this is total natural and you're not alone. The lack of desire can be caused by stress, pain, treatment side effects, how you feel about your body, the condition itself may also play a part and so much more.

However, if you enjoyed a healthy sex life before being diagnosed with a reproductive health condition, chances are you can still find pleasure in sexual intimacy. This is when being creative, thinking outside the box and redefining your sexual script comes in. You may find that intimacy and intercourse takes on a new meaning and you relate to your partner differently. Hugging, touching, holding, and cuddling may become more important, while actual intercourse may become less important.

Remember, it is important to communicate with your partner about your feelings regarding your sexual concerns. He or she cannot read your mind! Also, get as much information from your physician about your specific reproductive health condition. Also, consider working with a sex therapist or counseling to help answer any concerns you may have.

# CHAPTER 8:

# REMOVAL OF THE FEMALE REPRODUCTIVE SYSTEM

A hysterectomy is an operation to take out the uterus (womb), and sometimes the cervix and occasionally other reproductive organs. Although hysterectomy is the second most common surgery for women in the United States, that doesn't mean it's a breeze: the procedure can take a toll on the body. A hysterectomy can be done in several different ways, depending on your health history and the reason for your surgery. The different types of hysterectomy are:

- **Total hysterectomy** involves the removal of the uterus, including the cervix. The ovaries and the fallopian tubes may or may not be removed.

- **Supracervical hysterectomy** involves the removal of the uterus without the cervix. The cervix is the area that forms the very bottom of the uterus, and sits at the end of the vaginal canal.

- **Radical hysterectomy** involves removing the uterus, cervix, the tissue on both sides of the cervix, and the upper part of the vagina. A radical hysterectomy is most often used to treat certain types of cancer, such as cervical cancer.

- **Hysterectomy with oophorectomy and salpingoophorectomy. Oophorectomy** is the surgical removal of the ovary(s), while **salpingoophorectomy** is the removal of the ovary and the fallopian tubes. If the ovaries are not removed during the hysterectomy, a woman should not experience symptoms of menopause because the ovaries produce the hormone estrogen, which helps to manages symptoms of menopause. However, if both ovaries are removed during the hysterectomy, a woman will no longer have periods and may begin to immediately experience symptoms of menopause because hormone levels drop quickly without ovaries. In addition, the symptoms may be more intense than with natural menopause.

There are also many different procedures used to perform a hysterectomy. Usually the physician will decide which procedure you are the best candidate for based on reason for the hysterectomy, medical history, lifestyle, fitness level, job functionality, support system, etc. The different types of procedures include:

**Abdominal hysterectomy.** An abdominal hysterectomy is the most common type of hysterectomy. During this procedure, the doctor makes an incision in your lower abdomen, usually in the bikini area. The abdominal hysterectomy allows the whole abdomen and pelvis to be examined, which is an advantage in women with cancer or investigating growths of unclear cause. It also allows the physician easier access to remove the uterus and ovaries and fallopian tubes if needed.

**Vaginal hysterectomy.** A vaginal hysterectomy is involves removal of the uterus and the cervix, if necessary through a small incision at the top the vagina. If the cervix is not being removed, the incision is made around the cervix, which is then reattached when the surgery is finished. Women who have not had children may not have a large enough vaginal canal for this type of procedure.

**Laparoscopic hysterectomy.** A laparoscope is an instrument with a thin, lighted tube and a small camera that allows the physician to see the pelvic organs during the surgery. This special surgical tool is used to assist the physician in operating through small incisions in the abdomen and vagina. During a laparoscopic hysterectomy, the uterus is removed through the small cuts made in either your abdomen or your vagina. Laparoscopy-assisted vaginal hysterectomy (LAVH) is similar to the vaginal hysterectomy procedure described above, but it adds the use of a laparoscope. If a woman has such a history of prior surgery, or if she has a large pelvic mass, a regular abdominal hysterectomy might be considered.

**Robotic-assisted hysterectomy.** This minimally invasive hysterectomy involves the use of a robotic arm. The physician(s) use a computer to gently guide the surgical tools to remove the uterus, in tiny pieces, through small incisions in your lower abdomen. This technique is more accurate and precise utilizing the magnification of a 3-dimensional camera. The 3-D magnification enables the physician the ability to get into tiny spaces more easily and have a better view of the operation than with conventional laparoscopic surgery. The robotic-assisted hysterectomy is fairly new and requires specialized training on the robotic tools.

When deciding to have a hysterectomy, it is extremely important that you talk with your doctor about the different types of hysterectomies as well as the side effects, recovery and after care of the procedure. This will help you to make an informed decision based on your specific health care needs and/or concerns.

There are many reasons a woman may need to have a hysterectomy. Some reasons include:

- fibroids
- endometriosis
- heavy menstrual periods
- uterine polyps or endometrial polyps

Recovery time is based on the type of hysterectomy that you have. Generally, the least invasive hysterectomy procedure is likely to cause less pain and lose less blood than is typical with open abdominal surgery. Additionally, a woman is more likely to be able to resume normal daily activities more quickly than if she had an abdominal hysterectomy.

Most women are released from the hospital two to three days after having an abdominal hysterectomy; however, complete recovery takes weeks. Because vaginal and robotic hysterectomies are less surgically invasive than an abdominal hysterectomy, most women who have this type of procedure leave the hospital the next day. In some cases, a woman may be released the same day. The hospital will provide instructions regarding driving, bathing, and showering.

During the recovery period, plenty of rest is need to ensure that the body properly heals. It is not unusual to have a few cramps or feel a little bloated following a hysterectomy. Most women also have a bloody vaginal discharge after a hysterectomy that is normally a brownish color and may have a slight odor. This can continue for a few days to several weeks. It is important to refrain from housework and heavy lifting, 10 pounds or more, for the first few weeks. Increased movement and activity such as walking is encouraged. Abstain from sex or putting anything in the vagina, including tampons. It usually takes three to six weeks for a full recovery and return to normal activities, including sexual intercourse.

## SPEAKING OF SEX....

Over the years, having a hysterectomy has been synonymous with the end of sex. Virtually every woman expresses concerns; unfortunately, studies have shown that only half of gynecologists initiate a discussion of sex and few patients are brave enough to bring it up themselves. Sex is a vital part of life and the loss of sexual function can be devastating. I would not be completely honest if I said that sex life is not affected by having a hysterectomy.

Many women report a decline in arousal or vaginal lubrication or lack of intensity of orgasm. During a hysterectomy, some of the nerves, blood vessels, and ligaments are severed to remove the uterus. The uterus and its ligaments are rich sources of blood supply. As a result, sensation to the vagina, clitoris, and/or labia can be diminished. This loss of sensation can interfere with sexual functioning. Additionally because the uterus contracts during an orgasm, some women may notice the lack of sensation if they have previously experienced contractions.

If a woman has never experienced uterine contractions, then she will not notice the difference.

Desire and arousal may also be difficult for some women given the emotional connection some women experience because of hysterectomy. The psychological and physiological response to intercourse may be challenging for some women. The desire to have sex is based on a psychological response. Whenever there is a block/concern, it makes it difficult for a woman to become aroused. For example, as a result of having a hysterectomy, a woman may anticipate pain during intercourse. Or, because she has connected womanhood and sexuality with her uterus, the removal of her uterus may make her feel like less of a woman and less sexual, thus creating a loss of desire. The physiological response of arousal may be challenging after a hysterectomy given the lack of blood vessels in the genital area may make it difficult for a woman to become aroused. The lack of arousal and lubrication may make intercourse painful.

The decline in desire, arousal, and/or vaginal lubrication, which some women may experience after hysterectomy may also result from the removal of the ovaries. The ovaries produce the sex hormones estrogen, progesterone, and testosterone. Once the ovaries are removed, your body immediately stops producing estrogen and progesterone. Lubrication is lost and the vagina atrophies making sex painful which can contribute to loss of desire and/or arousal.

The changes to the vagina after hysterectomy can further hamper sexual function. The removal of the cervix requires that the vagina be shortened and sutured shut. This is called the vaginal cuff. The shortened vagina can present problems with deep penetration.

There is very little research and even less conversation regarding women's pre- and post-hysterectomy sexual functioning. How hysterectomy affects sexual function is not very clear and depends upon a number of internal and external factors. However, studies indicate that one of the most important facts that determines what sex after hysterectomy is like is what sex was like *before* hysterectomy.

Creating a sex life post-hysterectomy—as with pre-hysterectomy sex life—takes work, effort, and coordination. It's all about choreography! (See the section on sexual choreography in chapter 4.) Given that a normal—whatever that is—sex life takes work, one can only imagine how much effort has to go into creating an amazing post-hysterectomy sex life. Here are some helpful tips to help you enjoy sex post hysterectomy:

- **Become intimately acquainted with your body.** In order to experience pleasure, you have to be intimately acquainted with your body. Understanding your sexual response cycle (and how your body changes during each cycle) is the hallmark of sexual pleasure.

- **Communicate with your partner.** The first time you engage in intercourse after having a hysterectomy may be weird, so it is important to communicate with your partner. It is important to let your partner know if you are experiencing any discomfort or pain. Pain is an indication that something is not right with the body.

- **Start out slow.** Keep in mind that your body has undergone a major transition over the past few weeks; therefore, it is extremely important to take it nice and easy.

- **Engage in more foreplay.** Women need foreplay to help get their vaginal fluids flowing, lengthen the vagina, and help the body to relax.

- **Use more lubricant.** It is always a good idea to keep lubrication nearby. The more the vagina is lubricated, the less likely the lining the friction from intercourse will cause pain and/or ripping and tearing from intercourse. Rips and tears in the vagina help create a portal of entry for bacteria and other infections.

- **Change how you feel about sex.** Sex is more than physical. It is emotional, mental, spiritual, biochemical, etc. The mind and the body work together to optimize the sexual experience. Any negative attitudes, thoughts, or beliefs we have been taught regarding sexuality or our bodies can contribute to unpleasant sexual experiences.

- **Watch your position.** Certain sexual positions can cause pain during sex. Most positions that allow for deep, thrusting penetration can be painful for a woman, especially after a medical condition, medical procedure or if her partner is well endowed. Generally, positions that allow the woman to control the pace and penetration, e.g., woman on top, tend to be more comfortable for a sufferer of painful sex. In order to find out what works, experiment with different positions, techniques, and props (i.e., pillows) to find out the one(s) that offer the most stimulation with the least amount of pain.

Having a hysterectomy is just as much a spiritual, mental, emotional, biochemical, and social as it is physical, however it is not the end of life. Let's be clear: having a hysterectomy is *NOT* the defining factor for womanhood or sexuality — nor is having a hysterectomy a death sentence for your sex life. However, it is important to note that the recovery and healing experience for each woman will be different depending on a variety of factors such as support system, patient-physician relationship, medical history, thoughts, attitudes and beliefs, fitness levels, overall level of health, pain tolerance, medical adherence, etc.

To help with your recovery and healing, here are some additional helpful tips:

- **Do not try to be a superwoman.** Resist the temptation to work.

- **Accept the help**. Allow your family and friends to assist you with chores.

- **Listen to your body**. Do not over do it! Allow your body the time to heal properly.

- **Take medication (s) as prescribed** to stay ahead of the pain.

- **Get plenty of rest.** Remember you just had major surgery and your body is adjusting to the change.

- **Walk it out.** Get up and walk around after your hysterectomy as soon as you get permission to proceed from your doctor — even if you need assistance.

- **Wear comfortable clothes** that do not irritate your incisions.

- **Keep incisions clean and dry** so that they do not become infected.

- **Watch the kids, cats, and dog**. Sometimes kids, cats or dogs will just plop down unexpectedly. Keep a pillow on your stomach to protect your abdominal area.

- **Get support.** Talk to others who have had a hysterectomy. Not only is it a comfort to know that you're not alone, but you can also learn from others who had the same or similar procedure.

- **Just chill!** Enjoy your down time doing absolutely nothing at all!

Because many of the symptoms of reproductive health conditions, including sexually transmitted infections, can mimic each other and/or be misleading, it is extremely important that you speak with your physician(s) and/or sex therapist about your concerns. DO NOT try to diagnosis yourself! It may not be what you think and you can potentially end up doing more harm to yourself and your body.

In addition to the physical pain cause by a reproductive health condition, it is extremely important to also identify and address in mental, emotional, social, spiritual, biochemical, and/or relationship challenges that you may be experiencing. A reproductive health condition is nothing to be ashamed of or embarrassed about! The condition can be manageable if you are proactive and stay on top of your health. Learn all you can about your specific condition, work with a multi-disciplinary team of physicians and/or sex therapist to get treatment and communicate your needs to partner. You can still maintain a quality of life, as long as you are willing to go the extra mile to be an active participant in your treatment.

# CHAPTER 9:

# IMPORTANCE OF REPRODUCTIVE HEALTH CARE AND VULVOVAGINAL HEALTH

The conversation regarding women and girl's reproductive health rights is growing. More women and girls are become vocal and advocating for access to quality reproductive health care. Reproductive health care is fundamental to and inseparable from women's overall health and well-being. Access to affordable health services and to accurate, comprehensive health information are fundamental human rights. Improving reproductive and sexual health is crucial to eliminating health disparities, reducing rates of infectious diseases and infertility, and increasing educational attainment, career opportunities, financial stability, sustainable families and communities.

## PRESERVING OUR VULVOVAGINAL HEALTH

Women and girls vulvovaginal health is essential to life, not just her quality of life but the quality of further generations. Everyone in this world, was been born of a woman! We nurture the world in our womb, therefore how can be bring forth healthy generations with worn and rotten wombs Therefore it is extremely important to maintain a healthy reproductive system.

# Tips to Keep the Female Reproductive System Healthy

**To Douche, or Not to Douche…That is the Question**
Several studies have found that black and Latina women tend to use douches and feminine deodorizers more often than women of other races, making them more susceptible to higher rates of bacterial vaginosis and yeast infections. Douching is also more common among women of lower socioeconomic class, especially among white women.

Vulvas, like the rest of your body, can get messy. During puberty, the vagina starts to produce a fluid that can be white or clear and may leave marks on your underwear. Discharge is normal—it's your body's way of cleaning itself. The vagina also makes different types of discharge at various points in the menstrual cycle.

Sometimes people try to get rid of the natural discharge and smells of the vulva using douches. For years, women have been told to douche in order to feel fresher, cleanse their vagina, and keep it smell spring time fresh. This belief has been passed down throughout generations, and remains a common practice today. The only reason we are still caught up in the belief that douching is relevant is because the media and companies like Vagisil and Massengill have a product to market and sell. It is their job to make us to believe that the vagina is dirty and nasty, and in order to feel good about yourself and your vagina, you need to use products that will help the vagina smell like flowers. Having some vaginal odor and discharge is natural. However, if you notice a very strong or foul odor and/or a funny color discharge, it may be a sign of infection.

In recent years, however, many studies have shown that douching can actually be very harmful to the internal environment of the vagina. Douching can actually have adverse effects on the vagina by washing away healthy bacteria and pushing harmful bacteria further up into the vaginal canal. This can create an imbalance in the internal environment and make it much easier to get an infection.

The vagina is actually designed to cleanse itself. Washing the vagina with warm water is enough to keep clean. Using perfumed bath and body products only irritate the sensitive lining of the vagina as well as the inner and outer delicate folds of the vulva, the labia minora, and labia majora. Utilize caution when using a face towel or loofah on the vulva, especially dry ones, because they can carry bacteria that may be harmful to the vulva. If you must use a soap, stick to using a non-scented, alcohol-free soap only on the outside of the vulva area.

### Condoms, Dental Dams and Such

Making the decision not to wear a condom is like playing a game of Russian roulette — you never know when the bullet will hit you. Avoid the condom "cock-blocking" at all costs:

- "But I don't like using a condom!"
- "I can't feel it!"
- "I want to feel the REAL you!"
- "My dick gets soft when I put on a condom!"
- "What — you don't trust me? I'm clean!"

Just a few of the not-so clever-excuses one uses when it comes to condom aversion. Stop with the excuses and **wrap it up!** Would you rather find yourself explaining to a doctor why you have an itching, burning sensation with an icky drip coming from your penis, or perhaps why you have a foul-smelling discharge coming from your vagina? I think not! In lieu of abstinence, condoms are the best protection we have against STIs! In order to be effective, condoms should be used **consistently and correctly** for anal, oral, or vaginal sex. Condoms should only be used with a water-based or silicone-based lubricant, as this helps to reduce friction and chances of the condom breaking. **DO NOT use any oil-based lubricants such as massage oils, vegetable oil, Vaseline, or motor oil.** The oil will break down a condom in less than 60 seconds and now you are putting yourself as risk.

Additional Tips

- **Never go from anal sex to vaginal sex using the same condom.** If you do, you are increasing your possibility of getting an infection!

- **Avoid using novelty condoms**, such as glow in the dark condoms. Novelty condoms are just that, novelties. They are not intended for use in sexual activity.

- Condoms clog toilets! **Do not flush a condom down the toilet.** Throw away it in trashcan.

- **Never use a condom more than once.**

- **If the color of the condom is changed or uneven, do not use. If you have multiple partners, use a new condom with each one.**

- Condoms can also be used with sex toys, such as vibrators and dildos, to reduce risk of infections.

- **Stay away from the lambskin condoms!** Lambskin condoms are only good for preventing pregnancy.

- Store condoms in a cool, dry place (below 100° F) and avoid exposure to direct sunlight.

## ALL MEN DO NOT WEAR MAGNUMS!

Condoms come in sizes ranging from snuggies to extra-large! There is no one size fits all, although one size fits most! It is important to get the proper size, or else it may slip off or break during intercourse.

**Let's talk about dental dams**
What on Earth is a dental dam, Dr. TaMara?

So glad you asked! A dental damn is a thin, square sheet of latex or polyurethane used for oral-vaginal sex and oral-anal sex to help prevent the person's mouth from coming in contact with any bodily fluids.

During oral sex, dental dams should be placed between your mouth and the vagina. During anal sex, dental dams are placed between your mouth and the anus.

Dental dams should only be used one time and on one area of the body before being thrown away. You should never flip (or turn over) already used dental dams because this can result in the exchange of body fluids. Dental dams can also be used with lubricants for increased sensation. You can also put a bit of lubricant (non-oil-based) on the side of the dental dam that touches the skin to keep the latex from sticking. Dental dams also come in a variety of glycerin-free flavors to help with the taste.

Dental dams can be purchased from drugstores, online, community based organizations or aids service organization and from various public health departments. Unfortunately, many people report that dental dams may be hard to find, and they can be expensive. The good news though, is that dental dams are easy to make at home—all you need is a condom and scissors. So how do you make a dental dam?

### HOW TO MAKE DENTAL DAMS
- Unroll a condom. Make sure it has not expired!
- Cut off the tip very carefully
- Cut down one side of the condom
- Roll out flat

When making your own dental dams, it may be better to use a non-lubricated latex condom (as condoms lubricated with spermicide may taste bad or make your tongue numb). You can also choose to make dental dams from flavored condoms or from condoms and lubricants designed specifically for use during oral sex.

### Get tested for HIV together
If you and your Beloved are serious about taking your relationship to a sexual level, then consider going to be tested for HIV together. More importantly, go back a get your results together. When being tested for HIV, you may also want to consider being tested for other STIs. Some STIs,

such as chlamydia and gonorrhea are asymptomatic and may go undetected. Additionally, if a person has an STI, he or she is five times more likely to get a HIV. While being tested is great, it should not be your method of prevention. Changing behaviors that put you at risk for HIV, open and honest communication, and mutual monogamy should be your goal.

### Identify triggers

It is very important to learn what triggers your sexual responsiveness. For example, if you know that when you go out to the club you're likely to have a few drinks and end up leaving with someone to have sex, then the club is a trigger that you need to avoid and replace with a more healthy activity. Learning to identify what gets your hormones raging is essential to learning how to avoid those triggers and reduce your risk for HIV and other STIs.

### Change the type of sex you are having

Variety is the spice of life and we all like to break the monotony in the bedroom (or wherever you are having sex). However, the types of sex were having may be contributing to ones risk for HIV. Changing the type of sex you are having will also help to reduce your risk. Anal sex carries the most risk because the lining of the anus is thin and does not lubricate naturally causing it to rip and tear much easier. Vagina sex is the second most risky type of sex follow by oral sex. Keep in mind that the receptive partner is the partner that is most at risk because she or he is receiving the penis inside their anus or vagina. This increases their risk given the exposure to the fluid. **Here is an FYI: do not**

brush, floss, or engage in any activity that can cause a tear
or break in the lining of the jaw an hour or less before oral
sex, because it will increase the opportunity for HIV
transmission. If any semen or vaginal fluid gets inside of
your mouth, *swallow, spit, but do not let it sit!*

### Reduce the number of sexual partners

If you are a person that likes to engage in sex with multiple
partners, keep in mind that also puts you at multiple risks,
especially if the encounters are unprotected. Think of it this
way, every time you have sex with someone, you're having
sex with everyone that they have has sex with. Not only
does reducing the number of sexual partners lower your risk
for HIV, but it also lowers your risk for drama and other
indirect activities that put you at risk for HIV and other STIs.

### Hold up on the substances

We all have brought into the belief that alcohol makes the
sex better, heck even Jamie Foxx wrote a song about it
blaming it on the alcohol. Well contrary to popular belief
substances, prescription, legal or illegal, actually put you at
an increased risk for HIV and other sexually transmitted
infections. Anytime we over indulge in substances our
mental state becomes altered. Impaired judgement causes
you to make decisions that you would not normally make
such as having casual sexual encounters, because your
hormones are turned up. Substances can also impair motor
skills, which inhibit your ability to put on a condom and/or
dental dam (that is, if you can even think through the haze
of your buzz to even use one). In additional, substances can

control to erectile issues in men and vaginal dryness in women, which can contribute to more ripping and tearing during intercourse, creating a portal of entry for infections to enter the bloodstream.

**Take time to get to know your partner**

What's the rush—casual sex does not come without a cost and the cost could just be your life. Be sure to ask questions. With every sexual encounter, you must ask yourself "Is this orgasm is worth my life?" and "Am I willing to die for sex?" In essence, this is what you are saying when you fail to ask your sexual partners questions about his or her sexual past. Everyone has a sexual history. The number of partners is not very important, (because most people won't be honest anyway). You should be more consider with if he or she has had safer sex during **every single** sexual encounter. Additionally, questions to ask include:

- Have you been tested for HIV?
- Did you get your results?
- What were your results?
- Have you ever had a STI? If so, did you get it treated?

Heterosexual-identified individuals, you may also consider asking if your partner has ever engaged in any same sex sexual tryst. For lesbian or gay identified individuals, you may want to ask have you ever had sex with someone of the opposite sex. As difficult as it may be to ask these questions, it is very important to ask your sex partners about their sexual past. At the end of the day, *if you cannot ask your partner these questions, then maybe you should not be having sex with them!*

## Turn the lights on and open your eyes

You don't want to turn the lights on because you're concerned how your body looks or you want to be romantic. While having sex with the lights off can be less intimidating or be romantic, it can also be very dangerous. It is time to stop flip the switch and turn the light on and look at what you are getting yourself into. FYI, male condoms do not cover the testicles, vulva, or the perineum so if there are any genital warts or herpes lesions on any of those areas, you may be putting yourself at risk for transmission. In addition, you need to look at your sex partner's genitals to notice if there is any abnormal discharge coming out of the vagina or penis. If the lights are off and/or if you are not looking at your sex partner, how can keep yourself safe? Finally, when a person has one STI, it makes it much easier for them to get another, like five times, easier. Do not become a statistic because you are in the dark with your eyes closed.

## Learn to abstain

Your body is a temple! Not everyone deserves to receive your most precious gift. When you know your value and worth, you are less likely to do things to put yourself in danger. You respect yourself and your body. You are very cautious about whom you share yourself with. Every time you have sex with someone, you give a piece of yourself away that you cannot get back. There is an exchange of energy that remains with you; therefore, it is extremely critical that you are protective of the energy that you allow inside of your being. Finally, abstaining means abstaining from those "triggers" and substances that help to put an individual at risk for transmission of HIV/STIs.

## Take control of your sexuality

Don't allow love or your hormones to get the best of you. Make wise decisions regarding your sexual. Remember you are responsible for your sexual health. Women are sexually empowered and liberated but the sexual empowerment and liberation does not mean loose! Being sexually empowered and liberated means being in control of your sexuality, which includes your sexual desires and sexual expressions.

## Practice sexual exclusivity

Sexual exclusivity is similar to monogamy, in that it involves making the conscious decision to engaging in sex with only one person regardless of whether or not you are in a relationship. By practicing sexual exclusivity, you are reducing the number of sexual partners, which helps to lower risk for STIs and HIV.

## Don't forget about the lube!

Wetter is better, especially when it comes to sex. Vaginal lubrication is key to sexual pleasure for both men and women. Lubricant comes in a few forms: water-based, silicone-based and oil-based. Water- and silicone-based lubes are the best with condoms. Never use an oil-based lubricant with a condom — the oil will interact with the latex and cause it to break down. A good lubricant can go a long way in making sure that safer sex is pleasurable and fun. Lubricant is important in safer sex because it also makes condoms and dams slippery and less likely to break. Lubricants make safer sex feel better by cutting down on the dry kind of friction that many people find irritating

## How to Choose the Right Physician

Choosing a good physician to help manage vulvovaginal health is one of the most important health decisions you will make. The relationship with your physician can span decades. Physicians are often present and involved in caring and treating many aspects of your vulvovaginal health from birth to death and everything in between. It is an important job and should not be trusted to just anybody. There are many things to consider when trying to find the right physician: Do they

- demonstrate cultural humility?
- value bedside manner?
- demonstrate respect and compassion?
- have specialized training to treat your conditions?
- listen to you without interrupting?
- fully answer your questions?
- explain your diagnosis and treatment?
- offer treatment options in alignment with your values and belief systems?
- specify a date for a follow-up visit?
- have competent office staff?
- referral when scope of practice is beyond their expertise?

- provide patient-centered care?
- remain non-judgmental?
- include you as an autonomous agent and active participant in your care and treatment?

Additionally, you may want to make sure the doctor is in your insurance network, consider their hospital affiliations, research their credentials and expertise, and review patient satisfaction surveys before making your selection.

There is considerable healing power in the physician-patient alliance. Working together offers the opportunity to improve significantly the patient's quality of life and overall health status. Having a physician with whom you are comfortable seeing is truly an important objective. Like any other relationship, this one should be positive and add value to your life. It may take more than one visit for you and your new doctor to establish a comfortable relationship. If it doesn't happen, trust your instincts and find another. There are plenty of great physicians out there, so do your homework and make the choice that is right for you.

## Patient - Provider Relationship

The patient - provider relationship is essential to maintaining good

health. Research has shown that patients who have good relationships with their physicians tend to be more satisfied with their care and consequently experience better results. Additionally, physician's approach to the patient - provider relationship tends affect how engaged patients are in their health care. Trust and transparency forms the foundation of the patient-provider relationship. In order for the physician to make accurate diagnoses and provide optimal treatment recommendations, the patient must be able to confidently communicate all relevant information about an illness or injury to their physician.

## Routine Testing and Screenings

### PELVIC EXAM

The word "pelvic" refers to the pelvis. A pelvic exam helps a health care professionals evaluate the size and position of the vulva, uterus, cervix, fallopian tubes, ovaries, bladder, and rectum.

A pelvic exam also may be done to help detect certain cancers in their early stages, infections, including sexually transmitted infections (STIs), or other reproductive system problems.

Pelvic exams are usually performed: during a routine yearly physical exam, when a woman is pregnant, when a doctor is checking for an infection, and/or when a woman is having pain in her pelvic area or low back. Pelvic exams may also be used to determine the cause of abnormal uterine bleeding, evaluate pelvic organ abnormalities, such as uterine fibroids, ovarian cysts to collect evidence in cases of suspected sexual assault. Finally, a health care professional may conduct a pelvic exam before prescribing a method of birth control. Some methods of birth control, such as a diaphragm or intrauterine device, require a pelvic exam to make sure the device fits properly.

During a pelvic exam, you can expect to feel a little discomfort, but you should not feel pain during a pelvic exam. The exam itself takes about 10 minutes. If you have any questions during the exam, be sure to ask your doctor. A Pap test may also be done during the pelvic exam

<u>During a typical pelvic exam, your doctor or nurse will:</u>

- Ask you to take off your clothes in private (You will be given a gown or other covering.)

- Talk to you about any health concerns

- Ask you to lie on your back and relax

- Press down on areas of the lower stomach to feel the organs from the outside

- Help you get in position for the speculum exam (You may be asked to slide down to the end of the table.)

- Ask you to bend your knees and to place your feet in holders called stirrups

- Perform the speculum exam. During the exam, a device called a speculum will be inserted into the vagina. The speculum is opened to widen the vagina so that the vagina and cervix can be seen.

- Perform a Pap smear. Your doctor will use a plastic spatula and small brush to take a sample of cells from the cervix (A sample of fluid also may be taken from the vagina to test for infection.)

- Remove the speculum.

- Perform a bimanual exam. Your doctor will place two fingers inside the vagina and uses the other hand to gently press down on the area he or she is feeling. Your doctor notes if the organs have changed in size or shape.

- Sometimes a rectal exam is performed. Your doctor inserts a gloved finger into the rectum to detect any tumors or other abnormalities.

- Talk to you about the exam (You may be asked to return to get test results.)

When scheduling a pelvic exam, try to schedule the exam when you are not on your menstrual cycle, since blood can interfere with the results of a Pap test. However, if you have a new vaginal discharge or new or increasing pelvic pain, a pelvic exam may be done while you are having your period. Do not use douches, tampons, vaginal medicines, or vaginal sprays or powders for at least 24 hours. Do not have sex for 24 hours prior to the exam if you have abnormal vaginal discharge. No other special preparations are needed before having a pelvic exam. For your own comfort, you may want to empty your bladder before the exam.

If you have had problems with pelvic exams in the past or have experienced rape or sexual abuse, be sure to talk with your health care professional about your concerns or fears before the exam.

## PAP TEST

A Pap test, sometimes referred to as a Pap smear, is a method of cervical screening used to detect abnormalities in the cervical cells that may be potentially pre-cancerous and/or cancerous. Currently, a pap test is the best tool to detect precancerous conditions and hidden, small tumors that may lead to cervical cancer. If detected early, cervical cancer can be cured. Women should begin routine pap testing at the age of 18 or at the onset of sexual activity, if earlier, and continue screenings annually. After three or more consecutive satisfactory normal annual exams, the Pap test may be performed less frequently at the discretion of your health care professional. Screenings may be stopped for women over the age of 65 who have been adequately screened with normal results in the last 10 years and are not at high risk for cervical cancer. Most women ages 21 to 65 should get Pap tests as part of routine health care. Even if you are not currently sexually active, you should still have a Pap test. Women who do not have a cervix (usually because of a hysterectomy), **and** who do not have a history of cervical cancer or abnormal Pap results, do not need Pap tests.

The Pap test is normally done during a pelvic exam. A doctor uses a device called a speculum to widen the opening of the vagina so that the cervix and vagina can be examined. A plastic spatula and small brush are used to collect cells from the cervix. After the cells are taken, they are placed into a solution. The solution is sent to a lab for testing.

A normal Pap test means the cells from the cervix look normal. An abnormal Pap test means the cells do not look normal. In that case, further testing may need to be done to determine the cause for the abnormality i.e. cervical dysplasia. Pap tests can occasionally show signs of infection, but cannot be relied on to screen for sexually transmitted infections (STIs). Other tests are necessary to determine the presence of an STI.

There are several things you can do to help make the Pap test as accurate as possible. Avoid sex, douching, and vaginal creams for 48 hours before the test. In addition, do not schedule a Pap test during your menstrual cycle. The best time to be tested is 10 to 20 days after the first day of your period.

Regular Pap test screening, early detection and treatment of abnormal cervical cells is critical tool in finding and treating cervical cell changes before they progress to cervical cancer. If cervical cancer is suspected, your health care professional will proceed with additional testing.

**Activity: Using the Correct Terms with Physician**

Materials Needed
Journal to write down plan and any personal reflections about the activity

Directions
The next time you are at your physician's office, try using the medically accurate terminology to describe your body parts, symptoms, and sexual behaviors.

Journal questions to consider:
1. How did this activity make me feel?

2. Was it difficult to use the medically accurate terminology?

3. How did your physician receive the conversation?

4. How likely are you to continue using the medically accurate terminology?

Increase Your Vulvovaginal Esteem

There is a correlation between vulvovaginal health and low esteem. When we lack vulvovaginal esteem, we tend to place ourselves at risk because we are disassociated from our bodies and do not care enough to protect it. Low vulvovaginal esteem usually manifests itself in self-defeating behaviors. When we lack vulvovaginal esteem, we allow ourselves to be used and abused; seeking that which we believe is missing. Alternatively, we find comfort in sex, drugs, risky behaviors, and other unhealthy compulsions. Loving your body and knowing how your body works and what you are capable of helps to increase your confidence, your vulvovaginal esteem. The more confident you are, the more likely you are able to take care of your body, make better decisions, create stronger boundaries and facilitate healthier relationships. When you have high vulvovaginal esteem, you don't need someone else to validate you. This, unsurprisingly, leads to higher confidence. When you know your value and worth, you're less likely to do things to put yourself in danger — you respect yourself and your body, and you are very cautious about whom you share yourself with.

Activity: A Plan for Health, Wellness and Pleasure

## Materials Needed

Journal to write down plans and any personal reflections about the activity

## Directions

Using the activity: A Love Letter to Your Vulva, create a plan for health, wellness and pleasure.

As you create your plan, consider the following:

- How do you define health, wellness, and pleasure?
- What is your relationship like with your physician?
- How often do you go to the physician?
- How will you communicate with your sexual partner(s)?
- How will you break the cycle of how vulvovaginal health is discussed in your family? With you sister friends?
- How will you protect yourself for sexually transmitted infections?
- How will you reduce vulvovaginal irritation?

## Journal Questions to Consider

1. How did this activity make me feel?
2. What will I do with this health, wellness, and pleasure plan?
3. How committed am I to this health, wellness and pleasure plan?
4. How often will I review this health, wellness, and pleasure plan?

# CHAPTER 10: THE CHARGE

My Beloved!

This was all for YOU! I encourage you to go forth and share what you have learned with other women and girls. It is our responsibility to change the world by leaving a legacy of healthy, powerful, creative, dynamic, unapologetic empowered young women who embrace their vulvovaginal health!

No longer can we remain silent or stand by and allow women's reproductive health to be devalued. In order to change the trajectory, we must speak up and speak out! We stand up in solitary! Once we do, we will be to see a shift in our society that will begin to understand the investment in and the value of women's reproductive health!

Activity: A Love Letter to Your Vulva

Materials Needed
Journal to write down any personal reflections.

Directions
Write a love letter to your vulva.

Journal Questions to Consider

1. How did this activity make me feel?

2. In what ways have I been hurtful or harmful to my vulva and vagina?

3.  Where have I received my beliefs about my vulva and vagina?

4.  How have my beliefs and/or messages that I have received about my vulva and vagina helped to shape my attitude towards my body?

5.  How can I reshape my attitudes, thoughts, and beliefs about my vulva and vagina?

# ABOUT THE DR. TAMARA R. GRIFFIN

At age 13, Dr. TaMara Griffin told her mother that she wanted to be a sex therapist! Her passion is deeply rooted in providing individuals with the knowledge, tools, and skills needed to embrace their sexuality. Dr. TaMara is a certified clinical sexologist, sex therapist, author, speaker and radio host with more than 20 years experience speaking, writing and teaching about human sexuality. She travels the country speaking, consulting and providing extensive trainings to individuals, colleges, universities, business and other organizations about healthy sexuality. Dr. TaMara is the author of several books including: Live Inspired Feel Empowered, I AM Sex! A Comprehensive Guide to Understanding Women's Sexuality and It's Not The Birds And The Bees, It's Sex! How To Talk To Children About Sexuality. Dr. TaMara is also currently is the Editor in Chief for Our Sexuality! Magazine, the premiere magazine for women's sexuality and sexual health. She also is a freelance writer for many online magazines, social media websites or her personal blog "Live Inspired Feel Empowered." Dr. TaMara holds a Doctor of Philosophy (PhD) in Human Sexuality, Doctorate of Human Sexuality (DHS), Master of Social Work degree,  Master of Science degree in Education, and a Bachelor of Arts degree in Family Life Education. Dr. TaMara is certified in Clinical Sexology; and also a holds several additional certificates including: Sex Therapy, Clinical Sexology, and Erotology; just to name a few. Check out her radio show The Dr. TaMara Show every Friday on WBKE Vegas Radio at 4:00pm PST. Follow Dr. TaMara on all social media @drtamaragriffin.

# www.drtamaragriffin.com

www.ingramcontent.com/pod-product-compliance
Lightning Source LLC
Chambersburg PA
CBHW071350280526
45787CB00001B/277